SEX POSITIONS
FOR COUPLES

Table Of Contents

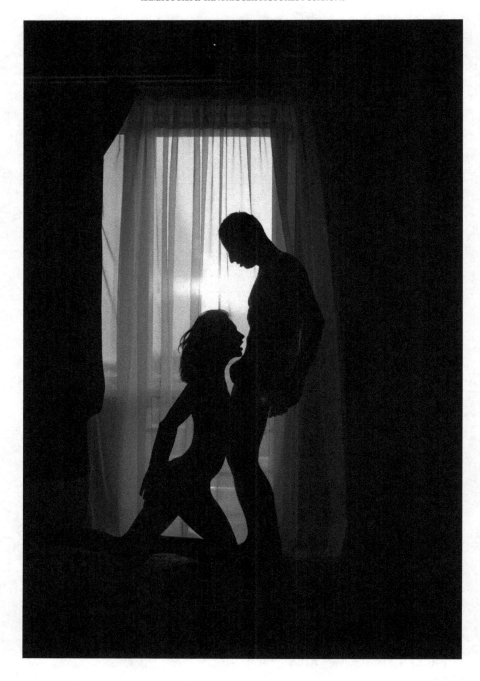

Introduction

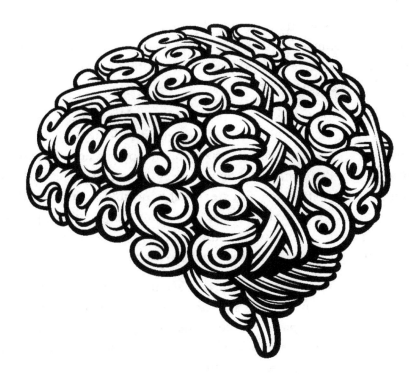

Other than orgasm, what could you consider the best thing concerning sex? There are numerous approaches to have it done: Upside-down, on the lounge chair, on a plane, from behind, generally, tenderly, the rundown goes on. Albeit conventional thoughts of manliness unjustifiably accept that all men are predominant in bed, incidentally, in real life, the sex positions men truly need are much more dynamic than you may suspect.

Everybody is diverse with regards to sexual inclinations, crimps, obsessions, and turn-ons. What's more, much the same as how somebody's vagina can influence how they accomplish a climax, factors like penis size — regardless of whether it's by-the-books enormous or more modest than normal — can essentially affect what positions turn out best for them. Although penis size isn't the main part of sex by far, it certainly becomes possibly the most important factor when you're attempting to sort out a position that feels better.

Consistency is something to be thankful for every now and then. There is something in particular about realizing you don't need to stress over something, that it'll just consistently be a similar way. Sex isn't really in agreement with that.

Getting into a sexual daily schedule in a romance is inescapable. We want what we want! In any case, inevitably, doing old stuff gets exhausting, and we as a whole realize what happens when sex with our spouse gets exhausting: the two players are crabby, baffled, and voraciously horny (to such an extent that your libido may even drop). The simplest method to escape a routine is, beyond question, attempting another position. It's the ageless method to make sex fun and energizing without truly testing all too much.

Sexual respites are ordinary in any event for the most energetic couples, and they may really be something to be thankful for. One clinician related a part of the issue to apathy: The passionate experience of weariness is difficult to overlook, and along these lines, it, in a way, enables individuals to lock-in.

The issue isn't the way that enthusiasm blurs, it's that we're so ill-equipped when it occurs. Hot sex is easy during the wedding trip period of a romance, and afterward, things unavoidably begin to chill. Most importantly, we're designed to crave for astonishment, assortment, and experience — and long haul connections are the specific inverse. Steadiness is the adversary of the amazement. Routine counterbalances assortment.

Organize sex as much as any piece of the romance and strive to bring back the assortment and novelty.

CHAPTER 1:

Revitalize Your Sex Life

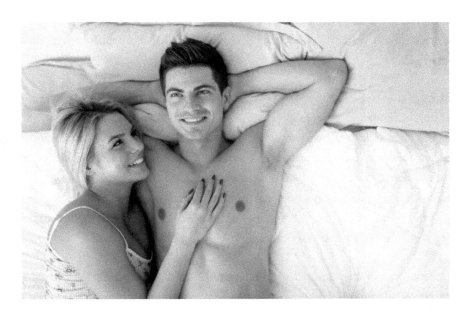

The vast majority of us can recall the hot and regular fiery minutes when the romance was new with our spouse. Be that as it may, ultimately, the fire of a decent love life may subside. After some time, the attractive nightie mopes are put away in the sock cabinet, the back-massage oil accumulates dust close to the competitor's foot powder in the medication box, and you and your mate have what feels like a modest sexual life.

Is your love affair with your spouse characterized more by kinship than enthusiasm, yet you actually love one another and haven't surrendered? Have confidence; it's normal for couples who have been hitched or focused on one another for some time and have occupied lives to float separated sincerely and explicitly. Fortunately, if you've lost the sparkle you once had, you can rediscover your romance and refocus.

The absence of sexual enthusiasm is the most widely recognized issue that carries couples to specialists, as per Marianne Brandon, creator of Unlocking the Sexy in Surrender. While each couple is unique, the most widely recognized situation you will see are couples with a forceful, passionate association, a mindful and deferential duty to each other — they like each other — however, they simply don't feel that sexual flash anymore.

During the beginning stage of a love life, numerous couples scarcely surface for oxygen because of the energy of experiencing passionate feelings. Shockingly, this delighted state doesn't keep going forever. Researchers have discovered that oxytocin (a bond hormone) is delivered during the underlying phase of fascination, which makes couples feel euphoric and turned on by actual friendship; for example, contacting and clasping hands. Oxytocin works like a medication, giving us quick rewards and restricting us to our sweetheart.

It's not unexpected to feel a feeling of dissatisfaction when our longing for sexual closeness doesn't coordinate with our spouses, and a distance is created. This is a typical battle among persevering couples adjusting occupations, nurturing, and closeness. Most sexual concerns originate from a relational battle in the marriage. One companion turns into the "follower" preferring closeness, and the other turns into a "distancer," preferring separateness. It's normal for the individual who is an enthusiastic distancer to need more sex and the other way around. For example, a few couples trade functions over a specific issue; for example, a lady who needs to be nearer genuinely to her significant other may not be keen on sex.

Let's be honest, when we become hopelessly in love and focus on somebody, we have high expectations that we'll feel euphoric and energized by the person in question uncertainly. This prompts unreasonable desires and frustration when the energy fades away. We figure sex will fill in recurrence and quality. However, within two years, 20% of love lives end up sexless (under 10 times each year), and an extra 15% experience low sex (under 25 times each year).

It's workable for couples to revive love by building a superior comprehension of themselves and one another and at last, developing a more grounded, more energetic association.

Did you realize that couples can likewise figure out how to revamp their minds to encounter more passionate and sexual closeness? The human mind, while brilliantly intricate, doesn't generally work to their greatest advantage, so they have to change up their sexual coexistence to encounter pleasurable emotions. Examination shows that we get a sound shot of dopamine (the feel-good hormone) when we are looking for remuneration and when there is something new to encounter. Likewise, fervor is adaptable, so the uplifted excitement that follows that state, a crazy ride, can be utilized to fire up your sexual coexistence.

- Examine your relationship. These incorporate ways you may be denying your spouse or going ahead too solid explicitly. Try not to reprimand one another and stop "habitual pettiness."

- Breakaway from the follower-distancer design. Distancers need to work on starting sex all the more regularly, and followers need to discover approaches to tell their mate "you're attractive," while keeping away from scrutinizing after sex.

- Resolve clashes handily. Try not to set aside feelings of disdain that can devastate your love affair. Encountering strife is inescapable, and couples who endeavor to maintain a strategic distance from it are in danger of creating stale connections.

- Boost up actual warmth. Actual contact discharges feel-good hormones. Clasping hands, embracing, and contacting can deliver oxytocin (the holding hormone) that lessens painfulness and creates a quieting uproar. Studies show that it's delivered during sexual climax and loving touch also. Real fondness additionally decreases pressure hormones — bringing down day-by-day levels of the pressure hormone cortisol.

- Allow good tension to pile up. Our cerebrums experience more delight when the expectation of the prize continues for quite a while before we get the real prize. Thus, take as much time as is needed, share dreams, change areas and make sex more passionate.

- Spend time with your spouse consistently. Attempt an assortment of exercises that bring you both delight. Have some good times seeking your spouse and work on being a tease. Remember to snuggle on the seat and give your spouse surprise kisses.

All things being equal, discussing issues with sexual closeness can, in some cases, exacerbate the situation. Thus, make a move and shake things up. Because your love life is experiencing a drought, it doesn't mean you are set out toward separation.

Make Dates

Couples that have been together for some time need to design time for sex. Make a date for sex. Try not to leave it alone as a reconsideration. Do whatever you like to do already, go out to see a film or supper, go for a stroll, have a glass of wine by candlelight, whatever the couple likes to do as a team. In short, put aside that time.

However, you may think, isn't booking dates for sex unromantic? Isn't sex expected to be unconstrained? Uncommon is the partner with an everyday organizer interest, all things considered.

What's the issue with making a date for sex? Individuals make arrangements for different things they appreciate, similar to ski excursions or meals out. I think the vast majority, particularly couples with kids, need to prepare because they, as of now, have such a great amount of stuck into their timetables. Of course, there are times when things suddenly fall together, yet those are upbeat mishaps.

Escape the House

One great proposal for a superior love life is to remove standard evenings from home. For couples that have been together for some time, sex can get normal. You're exhausted before the day's over after the work, the clothing, the children's soccer matches, and the tasks.

It very well may be difficult to surrender to the second when you're engaging in sexual relations in your all-around-recognizable room. Your brain meanders. Did I make sure to set the morning timer? What amount will it cost to fix that water harm on the roof?

Lovemaking is, generally, a current second encounter. The best sex comes when you're not pondering the past or the future, however just the present. Furthermore, that can be hard in a room where you've generally got grandmother's image grinning down on you.

Move away to a spot that is deprived of these tokens of regular day-to-day existence. It doesn't need to be a remarkable spot by the sea, or possibly it few out of every odd time. A non-descript place off the Interstate may be okay.

Redesign the Bedroom

Obviously, having a sexual coexistence that is completely subject to dates at inns and overnight sitters might be an issue in case you're not fantastically well off, childless, and jobless. Thus, notwithstanding a few outings away, roll out certain improvements at home. The room develops a lot of unremarkable affiliations. Yet, if you can successfully change your room into something new and extraordinary, that can have a major effect. What's more, a superior love affair doesn't need to introduce a spinning bed or roof mirrors. You don't have to accomplish something that will make the children or the maid go nuts.

Lighting a few candles is a conspicuous recommendation. However, perhaps getting a more pleasant arrangement of sheets and another blanket will have some kind of effect. Additionally, eliminating a portion of the garbage — the children's toys, the heaps of clothing — that will, in general, aggregate in a room can have an impact. Consider dumping the room TV as well, or possibly ignoring its existence for some time.

Sort Out What You Really Want

Everybody has sexual imaginations of some sort. In any case, for certain individuals, those imaginations can be covered pretty profoundly. On the off chance that your mate was to go to you this evening and state, "What's your definitive sexual imagination?" or "What would you like to change about how we have intercourse?" do you understand what you'd state?

In case you don't know, you're in good company. A few people need to accomplish a little work at sorting out what truly excites them. Yet, sorting out what you need is vital to having a superior love life.

Along these lines, give it a little exertion. There are a lot of instruments out there to help: books, magazines, recordings, etc. Whenever you've concocted a few thoughts, informing your spouse regarding them could be a diversion for both of you.

Discover What Your Spouse Wants

And afterward, there's the other side: You have to ask your spouse the very inquiries that you've asked yourself. What does your mate need from your affection life? One of the most well-known grumblings they hear is that one spouse needs to engage in sexual relations more than the other.

A few people may huffily accept that they simply have higher sex drives than their spouses do. However, perhaps your mate is searching for something else out of your affection life, yet hasn't felt ready to inquire. In this way, raise the subject. Talking transparently may carry you more like each other, and that is probably going to make sex additionally intriguing for both of you.

Take a stab at Something New

Taking a stab at something new in the room is a pretty clear recommendation for accomplishing a superior love life; however, it's one that numerous individuals experience difficulty following. For a lot of couples, the more they're together, the more they avoid any and all risks explicitly. You figure it would go the other way, but as individuals get more agreeable in a love affair, they have a sense of safety to attempt new things. Yet, that is not the situation.

Individuals oppose change, particularly cozy change. In case you're in a set-up romance, you may feel like you have more to lose. You would prefer not to cause trouble. Oppose the motivation to avoid any and all risks. This can mean a wide range of things — possibly undergarments, massage, sex toys, etc — and taking a stab at something new doesn't need to be over the top.

Individuals have a lot of insane ideas about what a sexual imagination should be. They figure it must mean sex on a Ferris wheel. Be that as it may, there are significantly fewer wild methods of trying different things with something new.

One little change that can have a major impact is to intrude on the example of how you, as a rule, engage in sexual relations. In case you're typically the bashful one who trusts that the other individual will start things, have a go at beginning it yourself. Simply face a challenge, regardless of whether it's somewhat one.

Try not to Ignore Problems

Sexual issues are a substantially more loosely held bit of information now than they used to be. For example, because of the endeavors of drug organizations and late-night funnies, there aren't numerous individuals left in the nation who don't know about prescriptions for erectile problems.

Obviously, that doesn't imply that each and every individual who needs assistance is getting it. Individuals who have sexual issues do frequently avoid sexuality since they would prefer not to confront disappointment. Yet, these issues should be tended to head-on.

Erectile brokenness has gotten the most consideration, yet there are a lot of different issues as well; for example, untimely discharge, a deficiency of charisma, or trouble arriving at climax brought about by meds or ailments

Ladies are approaching in bigger numbers and detailing sexual issues as well; for example, torment during intercourse or a failure to climax. Numerous ladies whine about vaginal dryness during sex, which can be agonizing.

Some sexual issues may require clinical consideration while others can be comprehended by attempting distinctive sexual strategies or purchasing a $5 jug of lube. Yet, the significant thing isn't to wade through with issues that are exacerbating your sexual coexistence. Try not to make do with an average sexual coexistence.

Proceed Gradually

A few couples find that the more they're together, the briefer and more efficient their sexual experiences can turn into. At the point when you move to another spot, you're continually evaluating various courses to get to the market or the tool shop. In any case, after time, you settle on the quickest course and just take that one. Not any more wandering. Something very similar happens to couples as they become more acquainted with one another explicitly.

In any case, the quickest, most effective course is certainly not what you need in the room. Zeroing in on the objective — and just the conspicuous pieces of the life systems — is the most noticeably terrible thing you can do. The best sex rises up out of the entire body's erotic nature — comfortable, energetic, innovative. It has no genuine heading; a tad bit of this, a tad bit of that.

Relaxed love production benefits everybody. Ladies get more turned on and appreciate sex more while men have fewer sexual issues and feel surer about themselves in bed. Everyone wins.

Try not to Worry About What Everyone Else Is Doing

One of the most widely recognized inquiries they get is, "What amount should we do it?" The inquiry suggests that the appropriate response is self-evident: more than I am, presently.

Inclining that you should be having a superior love life is most likely general. It clarifies the immense number of titles about sex in the self-improvement segment of the book shop and the consistency of articles about sex publicized on magazine covers at the checkout counter.

The way of life we live in — and particularly its movies, regardless of whether Hollywood passion or sexual entertainment — urges us to feel that we're not living up. So, how frequently "should" you have intercourse? There's no response to that. Quit attempting to choose how much sex you ought to have and choose the amount you need.

Continue Trying

Having a superior sexual coexistence will take some work. It resembles this: for some individuals, life is an unremitting guerilla battle with those additional 10 pounds that trap you when you're not focusing. Similarly, individuals can fall into a sexual trench, a "blah" love life, except if they're putting forth an attempt to keep things energizing.

You ought to expect that a few endeavors will crash and burn. A wound at a sexual pretend might be delivered absurdly by a badly coordinated call and aimlessly replying mail message from your relative. Or, on the other hand, perhaps the fragrant candles make you sniffle fiercely. Taking a stab at something new is continually putting you in danger of disappointment.

In any case, the significant thing is to continue attempting in any case. Try not to let reluctance make you avoid any and all risks. You ought never to acknowledge a simply normal love affair.

Man and Women's Sexual Behaviors

Sexual behaviors, any action — singular, between two people, or in a gathering — that prompts sexual excitement. There are two significant determinants of human sexual behavior: the acquired sexual reaction designs that have developed as a method for guaranteeing propagation which is a piece of every individual's hereditary legacy, and the level of restriction or different kinds of impact applied on people by society in the outflow of their sexuality. The goal here is to depict and clarify the two arrangements of components and their cooperation.

You should notice that restrictions in the culture of West and the youthfulness of the sociologies for quite a while obstructed exploration concerning human sexual behavior so that by the mid-twentieth century, logical information was to a great extent confined to singular case narratives that had been concentrated by such European authors such as Sigmund Freud, Richard, Freiherr (aristocrat) von Krafft-Ebing, and Havelock Ellis.

By the 1920s, nonetheless, the establishments had been laid for the broader measurable investigations that were led before World War II in the US. Of the two significant associations for sex education, one of them, the Institut für Sexualwissenschaft in Berlin, which was set up in 1897, was decimated in 1933 by the Nazis.

The second one, the Institute for Sex Research, started in Bloomington by the American sexologist Alfred Charles Kinsey at Indiana University in 1938, embraced the investigation of human sexual behavior. A significant part of the accompanying conversation lies on the discoveries of the Institute for Sex Research, which establish the most complete information accessible. The main other nation for which exhaustive information exists is Sweden.

Kinds of Human Behaviors

Human sexual behavior may advantageously be ordered by the number and sex of the members. There is singular behavior, including just a single individual, and there is socio-sexual behavior, including more than one individual. Socio-sexual behavior is commonly partitioned into hetero behavior (male with female) and gay action (male with male or female with female). On the off chance that at least three people are included, it is, obviously, conceivable to have straight and gay behavior at the same time.

In both single and socio-sexual behavior, there might be exercises that are adequately uncommon to warrant the name freak action. The term freak ought not to be utilized as an ethical judgment, however basically as demonstrating that such action isn't normal in a specific culture. Since human social orders contrast in their sexual practices, what is a freak in one society might be typical in another.

Single Behaviors

Self-masturbation is self-incitement to cause sexual excitement and, by and large, climax (sexual peak). Most masturbation is done in private as an end in itself, yet is in some cases rehearsed to encourage a socio-sexual love life.

Masturbation, by and large, starts at or before pubescence, is basic among guys, especially youthful guys; however, it turns out to be less incessant or is relinquished when socio-sexual behavior is accessible. Thus, masturbation is generally continuous among those yet to marry. Fewer females stroke off; in the United States, approximately one-half to 66% have done as such when contrasted with the vast majority of guys. Females likewise will, in general, diminish or end masturbation when they create socio-sexual connections. There is incredible individual variety in recurrence, with the goal that it is unfeasible to attempt to characterize what reach could be considered "ordinary."

The fantasy endures, regardless of logical verification unexpectedly, that masturbation is actually destructive. Nor is there proof that masturbation is juvenile behavior; it is basic among grown-ups denied of socio-sexual chances. While single masturbation gives joy and help from the strain of sexual fervor, it doesn't have the very mental satisfaction that communication with someone else gives; accordingly, incredibly couple of individuals favor masturbation to socio-sexual behavior. The mental noteworthiness of masturbation lies in how the individual respects it. For a few, it is weighed down with blame; for other people, it is delivered from strain with no passionate substance; and for other people, it is just another wellspring of joy to be appreciated for the good of its own.

Most guys and females have imaginations of some socio-sexual behavior while they stroke off. The imagination not rarely includes romanticized sexual spouses and exercises that the individual has not experienced and even may dodge actuality.

Since jerking off an individual is in sole control of the regions that are animated, the level of weight, and the quickness of development, masturbation is frequently more successful in creating sexual excitement and climax than is socio-sexual behavior during which the incitement is resolved somewhat by one's spouse.

Climax while sleeping obviously happens just in some people. Its causes are not entirely known. The possibility that it results from the weight of collected semen is invalid because not exclusively do nighttime emanations once in a while happen in guys on progressive evenings, however females experience climax while sleeping too. Now and again, climax while sleeping appears to be a compensatory wonder, happening during times when the individual has been denied of or avoids other sexual behavior. In different cases, it might result from outer boosts; for example, resting inclined or having late evening garments got between one's legs. Most climaxes during rest are joined by suggestive imaginations.

An extraordinary lion's share of men experiences climax while sleeping. This quite often starts and is generally continuous in youth, tending to vanish sometime down the road. Fewer females have climax while sleeping, and, in contrast to guys, they generally start having such experience when completely grown-up. Climax while sleeping is commonly rare, only occasionally surpassing twelve times each year for guys and three or four times each year for the normal female.

Most sexual excitement doesn't prompt sexual behavior with another person. People are continually presented with sexual improvements when seeing appealing people and are exposed to sexual topics in publicizing and broad communications. Reaction to such visual and other upgrades is most grounded in puberty and early grown-up life and normally step by step decays with propelling age. One of the important errands of growing up is figuring out how to adapt to one's sexual excitement and to accomplish some harmony between concealment, which can be damaging, and free articulation, which can prompt social troubles. There is extraordinary variety among people in the quality of sex drive and responsiveness, so this vital exercise of restriction is correspondingly troublesome or simple.

Socio-Sexual Behavior

By a long shot, the best measure of socio-sexual behavior is heterosexual behaviors between just a single female and a female. Heterosexual behavior oftentimes starts in adolescence, and, while quite a bit of it very well might be spurred by interest, for example, appearing or analyzing genitalia, numerous kids participate in sex play since it is pleasurable. The sexual drive and responsiveness are available in changing degrees in most kids and inactive in the rest.

With puberty, sex play is supplanted by dating, which is socially empowered, and dating unavoidably includes some actual contact, bringing about sexual excitement. This contact, known as petting, is a piece of the learning cycle, and eventually, of romance and the determination of a marriage mate.

Petting shifts from embracing, kissing, and summed up strokes of the dressed body, to procedures including genital incitement. Petting might be accomplished for the wellbeing of its own as a declaration of warmth and a wellspring of delight, and it might happen as a precursor to sex. This last type of petting is known as foreplay. In a minority of cases, yet a significant minority, petting prompts climax and might fill in for sex.

Barring foreplay, petting is usually generalized, starting with embracing and kissing and bit by bit heightening to incitement of the bosoms and genitalia. In many social orders, petting and its heightening are started by the male more regularly than by the female, who by and large oddballs or acknowledges the male's suggestions, however, shuns assuming a more forceful job. Petting in some structure is a close general human experience and is important in mate choice, as well as a method for figuring out how to connect with someone else explicitly.

Intercourse, inserting the penis into the female's vagina, is seen by society distinctively relying on the conjugal status of the people. Most human social orders grant early copulation in any event in specific situations. In more oppressive social orders, for example, present-day Western culture, it is bound to be endured (however not energized) if the people plan marriage. Conjugal sex is normally viewed as a commitment in many social orders. Extramarital intercourse, especially by spouses, is commonly denounced and, whenever allowed, will be permitted uniquely under extraordinary conditions or with determined people.

Social orders will, in general, be more merciful toward guys than females concerning extramarital sex. This twofold norm of profound quality is likewise observed in early life. Post-marital copulation (i.e., intercourse by isolated, separated, or bereft people) is quite often overlooked. Indeed, even social orders that attempt to keep intercourse to marriage perceive the trouble of attempting to constrain forbearance upon explicitly experienced and generally more established people.

In the United States and quite a bit of Europe, there has been, inside the only remaining century, a reformist pattern toward an expansion in early intercourse. As of now, in the United States, at any rate, 75% of the guys and over a portion of the females have encountered early intercourse. The extents for this experience change in various gatherings and financial classes. In Scandinavia, the rate of early copulation is far more prominent, surpassing the 90% imprint in Sweden where it is currently anticipated behavior.

Extramarital sex keeps on being transparently censured, however, is turning out to be more endured furtively, especially if moderating conditions are included. In certain zones, for example, southern Europe and Latin America, extramarital intercourse is anticipated from most spouses and is acknowledged by society if the behavior isn't excessively blatant. The spouses don't, for the most part, affirm yet are surrendered to what they accept to be a manly affinity. In the United States, where, at any rate, a large portion of the spouses and one-fourth of the wives have extramarital copulation sooner or later in their lives, there have as of late grew little associations or clubs that exist to give extramarital intercourse to wedded couples.

Despite the exposure they have caused, be that as it may, amazingly, a couple of people have had a place with such associations. Most extramarital intercourse is done subtly without the information on the living spouse. Most married couples feel possessive of their lifemates and decipher extramarital behavior as a maligning on their own sexual sufficiency as showing a deficiency of fondness and similar to a wellspring of social disfavor.

People are not characteristically monogamous yet have a characteristic longing for variety in their sexuality as in different parts of life. A few social orders have given delivery to these cravings by suspending the limitations on extramarital intercourse on unique events or with specific people, and in present-day Western culture, a specific measure of extramarital tease or mellow petting at parties isn't viewed as surprising conduct.

Conversation of socio-sexual behavior would be inadequate without some note of the job it has played in service and religion. While the significant religions of today are to shifting degrees anti-sexual, numerous religions have joined sexual behavior into their rituals and functions. Individuals' old and proceeding with interest in their own richness and in that of food plants and creatures make such an association among sex and religion inescapable, especially among people groups with unsure food supplies.

In many religions, the gods were considered to have dynamic sexual lives, and now and again took a sexual interest in people. In such a manner, it is critical that in Christianity sexual behavior is missing in paradise and sexual proclivities are attributed uniquely to fiendish extraordinary creatures: Satan, fallen angels, incubi, and succubi (spirits or evil presences who search out dozing people for sex).

Regardless of whether a conduct is deciphered by society or the person as suggestive (i.e., equipped for inducing sexual reaction) relies predominantly upon the setting where the behavior happens. A kiss, for instance, may communicate agamic friendship (as a kiss between family members), regard (a French official kissing a warrior in the wake of presenting a decoration on him), or veneration (kissing the hand or foot of a pope), or it very well might be an easygoing welcome and social convenience. In any event, something as explicit as contacting genitalia isn't interpreted as sexual whenever accomplished for clinical reasons. All in all, the obvious inspiration of the behavior decides its translation.

People are incredibly delicate in deciding inspirations: a welcome kiss, whenever extended over a second or two, takes on a sexual undertone, and ongoing examinations show that if a grown-up male at a gathering stands nearer than the length of his hand and lower arm to a female, she, by and large, attributes a sexual rationale to his vicinity. Bareness is interpreted as sensual or even as a sexual greeting — except if it happens in a clinical setting, in a gathering comprising of yet one sex, or in a nudist camp.

The Importance Of Intimacy

Closeness normally means common weakness, receptiveness, and sharing. It is regularly present right up front, cherishing connections; for example, romances and companionships. The term is additionally some of the time used to allude to sexual connections, however, closeness doesn't need to be sexual.

Closeness can be indispensable to keeping up a solid public activity. If you stay away from closeness, you may end up secluded or in a consistent clash with others. At the point when the dread of closeness upsets a love life, couples guiding or singular treatment may help.

The Cambridge word reference characterizes closeness as 'the condition of having a nearby close to a home love affair with somebody.' It is the inclination of being associated with someone else from the heart, psyche, and soul. Two individuals can be supposed to be intimate when they feel close and agreeable enough to show each other their weak sides and offer each other's carries on with everything. They share regular dreams and desires and become each other's wellbeing nets.

At the point when two spouses are youthful, and the romance is new, there is huge loads of sexual closeness. With time, sex starts to assume a lower priority, and with that, separation starts to sneak in. A passion for being 'underestimated' grabs hold in the romance. As the obligations of children, maturing guardians, dealing with a home and money takes the front seat, a couple's romance gets pushed to the botton. This is when couples whine the most about an absence of closeness in their connections.

Notwithstanding, that is because most couples befuddled the absence of sex as a nonappearance of closeness. Given that there are various kinds of closeness in love life, this can be viewed as too thin a view. While these different types of closeness may effectively be there in your love life, it is conceivable that you haven't remembered them yet attributable to cultural development that compares closeness with an actual association alone.

Closeness is significant in light of the fact that people are social animals who blossom with close-to-home associations with others. While closeness hints at pictures of passionate connections, it can likewise happen in dear fellowships, parent-kid connections, and siblinghood.

Various individuals have diverse closeness needs. One spouse may feel the requirement for more closeness while the other one feels that their love life is okay. Nonetheless, on the off chance that one of you has an issue, at that point, the love affair has an issue. In a sound love affair, the two individuals should feel cheerful and fulfilled.

The main thing more terrible for a romance than not being personal enough is constraining more noteworthy closeness. Much the same as certain individuals have various requirements for closeness; various individuals fill in closeness at various rates.

If you are prepared for more closeness with your mate, disclose to them that. Nonetheless, you ought to likewise have the option to show restraint toward them and ensure that you're not moving excessively quick for them or making them awkward. Getting cozier with somebody can be hard for certain individuals, and you have to give them time.

On the off chance that your spouse wants to be more private, you have to regard their desires, regardless of whether you don't feel the need yourself. Tell your spouse that you are eager to work with them on building closeness yet, in addition, clarify your present limits. You should be eager to open up to your mate and attempt new things with them, yet your spouse ought to likewise be willing and ready to require some serious energy getting more personal with you without causing you to do things that you don't care for or that cause you to feel awkward. Since we have gone to a comprehension of how closeness is significant, by what method can you and your spouse create closeness in your marriage?

Sadly, we as a whole come into associations with things, and for certain individuals, the stuff is so convoluted or so disturbing that it's hard for them to be personal. For a few, their troubles with trust, responsibility, or weakness are established in youth closeness and trust issues. However, because it's hard, it doesn't mean it's not something all couples ought to make progress toward.

For what reason would it be a good idea for you to develop closeness in your love affair? Not exclusively does closeness incredibly profit your marriage; it additionally benefits your physical and emotional well-being. Peruse on to find out about some extra advantages of an incredible sexual coexistence.

- Intimacy Improves Your Physical Health

A functioning sexual coexistence is an acceptable exercise as a 30-minute sex meeting can consume anyplace between 70-150 calories. (This is comparable to going for a short stroll.) Likewise, substantial breathing builds your oxygen consumption, which is valuable for both mental and actual wellbeing. It can assist you with remaining fit as a fiddle and furthermore do ponders for your temperament.

- Intimacy Relieves you from Stress

Like any actual behavior, sex is an incredible method to soothe pressure. During sex, the body feels loose, and a synthetic called oxytocin is delivered during the climax. Oxytocin is useful for your physical and emotional wellness. Oxytocin is additionally the motivation behind why numerous individuals feel languid and loose after peaking. In any case, sex isn't the best way to deliver oxytocin. You can likewise trigger this synthetic while embracing, snuggling, or by and large, being loving with your mate.

- Intimacy Makes Your Love Life Stronger

A love life without physical, as well as passionate closeness, is destined to be fruitless. Over the long run, as the two individuals become progressively detached, it turns out to be anything but difficult to cheat or leave the romance when they look for closeness somewhere else. Men normally search for physical closeness while ladies need passionate association.

We as a whole have an innate need to feel cherished and increased in value by our critical others and seeing each other is the establishment of any strong romance. It gives the two spouses a conviction that all is good and certainty when they realize they have each other for help regardless of what comes up.

At the point when these key fixings are missing, it gets hard to assemble and keep up a close connection. In this way, it bodes well that developing closeness reinforces the romance. At the point when the two spouses have a sense of security and are associated, it makes a positive cycle that bonds the couple together in expanding levels of closeness.

- Intimacy Boosts Your Self-Confidence.

Self-assurance is significant for any individual, paying little mind to age or romance status. At the point when men are denied sex and association, it can bring about an absence of self-assurance. Likewise, ladies can feel genuinely shaky and contemplate whether there is a major issue with their appearance. This is another motivation behind why closeness is fundamental in a love affair. An absence of fearlessness can be harmful to the two people, and it can negatively affect their everyday lives.

- Intimacy Gives You a Longer Life.

Sex has been connected to numerous medical advantages. Did you realize it can assuage constant painfulness? This is because sex discharges endorphins, which help in calming torment. Next time you get cerebral pain or a headache, consider engaging in sexual relations before going after the jug of Advil. Ladies have additionally discovered sex to help with feminine spasms and joint pain.

Besides, ordinary sex forestalls or brings down the danger of some cardiovascular illnesses like strokes and elevated cholesterol levels. During sex, the body gets cardiovascular exercise, which adds to a solid heart. Sex brings down your circulatory strain, causes you to rest better, and has even been connected to diminished danger of prostate malignancy! Engaging in sexual relations in any event once seven days can likewise help your insusceptible framework. A solid invulnerable framework lessens the danger of ailment and other actual infirmities. To put it plainly, sex can assist you with living a more extended, more advantageous life!

- Intimacy Helps Women to Regulate Their Hormone Levels.

Ladies experiencing misery and ongoing pressure, as a rule, have unpredictable periods. Sex can help as it improves temperament by offsetting hormone levels. Likewise, it helps fruitfulness in ladies and can forestall issues like pelvic painfulness. Notwithstanding the actual advantages, feeling adored, secure, and cheerful assumes a significant part in lessening feelings of anxiety in ladies.

- Intimacy Can help You with Blood Circulation.

Blood flow is critical to your general wellbeing. It keeps you from getting sick, and it improves your dozing designs and your temperament levels. Sex is a simple method to expand your blood dissemination, improving the stream to your organs and cerebrum while assisting with lessening circulatory strain.

- Sex Makes Your Bones and Muscles Stronger.

Sex fortifies muscles and bones, particularly in men, as it helps the creation of testosterone, which assumes a significant function in the psychological and actual soundness of men. It likewise builds the moxie, which thus drives men to look for closeness.

In light of these models, plainly closeness and sex assume a critical function in keeping you solid and glad genuinely, intellectually, and inwardly. So, what happens when you're feeling the loss of that critical fixing in your marriage?

Emotional Intimacy

At the point when you consider closeness in a love affair, it's conceivable that your contemplations hop first to the physical. Be that as it may, building passionate closeness is, in actuality, similarly significant. At the point when mates need passionate closeness, it very well may be hard to sympathize with one another and construct trust. Fortunately, in case you're uncertain whether you're there yet, romance specialists can assist you with searching for signs.

Emotional closeness is an ability, yet it, in the end, turns into a method of being in a love affair. It includes a degree of receptiveness and weakness from the two individuals and expands the general feeling of closeness we feel with our spouses in everyday life. Without emotional closeness, it very well may be difficult for couples to face the hardships of coexistence.

Emotional closeness is, at last, the magic that binds a love life after the underlying energy misfires. Couples who are genuinely private can conquer struggle all the more effectively because they see each other better and can convey their emotions to one another. Fortunately, there are approaches to manufacture emotional closeness if you haven't exactly taken advantage of it yet. To start with, you have to monitor your love affair.

Passionate closeness is so significant for our individual prosperity, just as the wellbeing of our love affair. Stressors, change, plans, actual separation, mental distraction, the back and forth movement of life are endless things that can prompt our getting up one morning and feeling removed from our personal other.

If we consider closeness a level of special association, we understand that even great things occurring in our lives can prompt diminished closeness. All things considered, regularly great changes or individual accomplishments additionally involve profound ventures for exercises that don't really incorporate our spouses. Models incorporate an advancement at work or helping a companion through a difficult stretch.

On the off chance that you incline that you and your mate could utilize a closeness help, here are good thoughts for firing up an association that needs reestablishment or is only due for some tender loving care.

How to Improve Emotional Intimacy
Lacking passionate closeness is a typical test in passionate connections. For instance, you and your spouse may find that it's harder to trust one another than it used to be. Or then again, you may feel detached, regardless of whether you hobnob. Closeness difficulties may particularly emerge in specific situations — on the off chance that you've been together for quite a while, for example, or if you've as of late experienced a major life change (like moving or beginning a new position) that saps your energy.

Yet, building emotional closeness doesn't need to include significant changes. Evaluate the accompanying little everyday practices to revive your bond and feel nearer than any time in recent memory.

- Be understanding.

Getting to genuinely understand somebody is a real responsibility. The trust-building measure is frequently a moderate one. Closeness isn't a race.

- Start with the simple stuff.

If you think that it's simpler to discuss the future than the past, at that point, start by sharing your fantasies and objectives. As trust fabricates, you may think that it's less terrifying to discuss the more troublesome subjects.

- Talk straightforwardly about your requirements.

Is it accurate to say that you are somebody who needs a ton of time alone to revive? How frequently do you like to engage in sexual relations? You can forestall plenty of misconceptions if you tell your spouse sincerely what you need as opposed to accepting your longings are "self-evident."

- Respect each other's disparities.

Indeed, even the most private mates actually have their own characters. You and your spouse don't have to concur on everything to cherish one another.

- Be deliberately powerless to procure their trust

Even on the off chance that we've invested a gigantic measure of energy with somebody, it's occasionally hard to separate our own dividers. Although you can't constrain the other to get defenseless, you can make a special effort to be weak yourself.

The practice of key weakness is fundamentally significant. Rather than attempting to be helpless in each aspect of your life, pick one spot to begin.

This may mean sharing something that occurred at work; you probably won't have in any case examined, communicating an inclination you've had in the past that has been difficult to share, or uncovering a reality about yourself that you've been clutching.

- Give your spouse everyday certifications and praises

Whether you're a half year into a love story or 60 years profound, it's anything but difficult to underestimate our mate's positive ascribes and some of the time hard to communicate the amount we esteem them.

Making a propensity for offering explicit commendations and confirmations to your spouse can assist you with keeping your point of view regarding why this individual is extraordinary to you, and it can assist them with realizing you see them. You never need your spouse to feel imperceptible because you neglected to share your appreciation.

These verbal insistences can be as straightforward as saying, "I need you to know how profoundly I love you" or "I truly like the effort you've put into doing X."

- Prioritize sexual fulfillment

A study distributed in the Journal of Sex and Marital Therapy found that couples announced having a more prominent passionate association when they were explicitly fulfilled. In that sense, the two are inseparably connected. While engaging in sexual relations itself isn't a fix just to improve your passionate bond, setting aside the effort to learn and investigate your mate's longings — and having the equivalent responded — can prompt more noteworthy passion of emotional association all through the room. Make an effort to break out of your everyday daily schedule

With how bustling life gets, it's anything but difficult to hit a safe place level in which we move past one another, basically attempting to scratch things off our daily agendas. This is a distinct difference from the start of a romance, when all that we do appears to be new and energizing, and when we exceed all expectations. This can imply that we have dismissed the benefit of getting things done for one another that creates happiness or closeness in the other individual. We quit attempting to dazzle, we quit attempting to comprehend, and in such conditions, weakness and passion can get lost to the daily schedule of the ordinary. It is unfathomably significant that we set aside a few minutes for one another in a more significant manner than just supper or sleep time together. Garner motivation from those early seeking days in a love affair. Possibly you plan unconstrained fledglings square moving night out on the town; you choose to go for frozen yogurt and a walk, you appear with "because" blossoms, or you plunk down together and plan an end of the week escape.

- Make time together to plan something significant for the both of you

Of course, a night out is significant. Yet, on the off chance that it's a formal occasion where you go out and sit opposite one another in a corner browsing email on your smartphone or talking about the most recent ludicrous thing your kid attempted to pull off at school, you're not developing your association. Association developing exercises get you zeroed in on one another as individuals — and on your romance. Take a picturesque drive to get frozen yogurt, clean the tub together, or take a cooking class. Working through the standard stressors in a more pleasant setting like an eatery isn't any way that is better than working through the stressors over the kitchen table regarding to building closeness.

- Be interested

Regularly, because we become put resources into the rightness or accuracy of our conclusions, we quit being interested regarding why the other individual feels how they do about a given issue. Valuing the why of where your cozy spouse is coming from — without feeling undermined that their for what reason may best yours — is a ground-breaking method for building compassion (without offering up your own input), and sympathy is profoundly private. Putting forth the attempt to comprehend someone else doesn't submit you to concurring with them; it does anyway exhibit a profound level of caring even with regards to a contradiction.

- Be accessible in some other manner

To immediately infuse closeness into your love life, settle on the choice to be accessible to your spouse in a manner you, for the most part, are definitely not. Not because you ought to or because you owe it to them, but since you can. Make them happy by consenting to deal with a task you normally fight/stay away from; offer to go with them on something you, as a rule, take a pass on; or astonish them with something they care about, making a most loved feast or watching that film they love, and you can't stand while you nestle. The generosity of surprise boosts intimacy greatly.

- Make a list. A "Nice" One

It's anything but difficult to get zeroed in on one another's defects, and there will consistently be a lot of them. Take a stab at plunking down separately or with your mate and making appreciation or "pleasant" records, enumerating however many things as could be expected under the circumstances that you acknowledge or potentially appreciate about your spouse. Regardless of whether you do it all alone, it will assist you with pulling together on purposes of association what attracted you to them at first and paying little heed to all the disturbances we unavoidably face throughout close connections.

- Put resources into yourself

Numerous astute masterminds have seen in various manners that two resilient people together make for a more grounded romance. Putting resources into yourself, your wellbeing, and your self-awareness are a significant piece of your well-being as a team. At the point when you are feeling your best, and in contact with how you are thinking and feeling, you can partake all the more completely, carefully, and genuinely. Invest some quality energy with yourself. Have significant discussions with loved ones, ensure you are being devoted to your needs, and continue searching for approaches to develop into who you are as a person.

- Be bold, not forceful

Shirking decimates closeness. On the off chance that you and your spouse are commonly or separately evading a difficult subject that should be tended to, you are gradually destroying your association. Now and then, significant points must be postponed for a suitable time and spot, yet long haul shirking resembles wind and water on stone — the unpretentious changes may not be observable on an everyday premise except one day, a huge disintegration will be clear. The weakness needed to begin a troublesome discussion that should be had is a critical driver of closeness. It imparts to your mate that you put resources into the strength of the love story than evading individual uneasiness.

- Practice non-critical tuning in

It might sound basic; however, you can up the closeness of even short discussions by putting forth an attempt to truly tune in to your spouse. We're so used to laying our own decisions, contemplations, and presumptions on top of our own or others' musings and activities.

At the point when we're too bustling tuning into the foundation commotion of judgment and considering what to state straight away, it very well may be truly hard to remain zeroed in on what your spouse is attempting to impart. You're passing up a great deal of key data. In addition to the fact that you miss the words, this individual is stating, however, how they are stating it also.

Practically speaking, non-critical listening can mean evaluating the accompanying abilities: Nodding and keeping in touch while your mate talks to flag that they have your complete consideration. Resisting the inclination to turn the discussion toward yourself; for instance, you may pose explaining inquiries rather than leaping to your own insight. Leave space for quietness; now and again, remaining calm can give your spouse space to share all the more profoundly.

- Offer thanks for the easily overlooked details

Offering thanks for your spouse goes past trying to say "I love you"— it can likewise mean sharing your gratefulness for all the seemingly insignificant details they do every day. Have a go at saying a straightforward "thank you" for things you normally underestimate. Perhaps your mate made sure to purchase toothpaste, or possibly they got up to turn off the light you left on in the other room. These little signals are large demonstrations of mindfulness, and effectively recognizing them can remind you both how profound your association goes.

- Humor each other's interests

Developing your own individual advantages is significant in any love affair; however, it very well may be similarly imperative to show interest and eagerness for the things your dearest loves.

For instance, does your spouse have a most loved book you've never perused? Perusing it can give you new knowledge into what really matters to your spouse, and setting aside the effort to do so is an incredible method to exhibit warmth. It additionally gives you a mutual encounter to examine.

Or then again, perhaps your mate has a most loved diversion — climbing, playing the guitar, heating — that you don't think a lot about. Have a go at requesting that they assist you with studying it. You will investigate another side of your spouse, in addition to you may end up with a fun new shared behavior!

- Have a go at something new together

You can likewise evaluate a spic and span experience together. Exploration has demonstrated that trying new exercises together can help revive closeness for long-haul spouses.

This may be as straightforward as evaluating another eatery together, pursuing a salsa dance or cooking class you're both intrigued by, or investigating another piece of the city. Or on the other hand, you may find that there's another side interest you both need to engage in, such as joining a games association or a melodic gathering.

In any of these cases, diving in together can give you a novel method to associate and a wellspring of energizing shared recollections.

- Change your landscape

Similarly, visiting another spot together can stir up your romance and give you another feeling of closeness. A get-away together is the most evident approach to do this, yet if a major excursion isn't in the cards at present, there are still loads of different ways you can pick up the advantages of a change in landscape.

Have a go at thinking about your own town or city how a traveler may: are there exhibition halls, destinations, or different attractions that you've never visited? Shouldn't something be said about close-by objections close enough for a road trip? On the off chance that, for instance, you both live in New York City and you've never been to the Statue of Liberty, think about creating a trip of it.

You can even attempt this in your own home — reworking a room together, or going through the day on the terrace when you, as a rule, sit on the sofa, can be a startling method to cause your romance to feel somewhat fresher.

- Address closeness issues in couples their singular therapy or individual counseling

If you locate that an absence of closeness is a reliable issue for you, as well as your mate, think about observing an advisor for additional help.

In couples directing, you can rehearse successful relational abilities, get an uphold around building closeness and work on any hidden issues that may make it harder to associate.

In individual treatment, you can handle feelings identified with closeness, gain knowledge into what may make closeness hard for you, and practice systems for interacting all the more intimately with your spouse.

Physical Intimacy

Physical closeness reinforces the connection between two individuals and cultivates closeness, love, and fondness between couples. It is a significant folio that assists couples with resolving the contrasts between them. Physical closeness constructs a more grounded association between two individuals by moderating any current pessimism. Oxytocin, a hormone and a synapse delivered during the private minutes between the couples, upgrades trust and a more grounded feeling of friendship between couples. These are actually private methods more than basically going to the room with your companion. Physical closeness can go from eye to eye connection, clasping hands, nestling, and obviously, sex. Physical closeness includes a profound, passionate association that is fortified when you are in close erotic nearness to your mate. Contacting, both impractically and something else can help reinforce this bond. Having this profound bond can positively affect essentially every other part of your love life.

Physical closeness in a love story is a significant standard for some couples — and it's not just about sex. There are likewise exercises that include actual touch, such as clasping hands, rubs, and in any event, being loosened up enough to toss your legs on top of your spouse's while you're viewing a film. What's more, it's significant that you're getting enough physical closeness in your love affair.

Concerning the amount you should be contacting, there's no bar to quantify yourself against. All things considered, it's about what works for you and your mate. I think this is an extremely close-to-home thing that fluctuates from couple to couple. The main problem isn't whether there is sufficient physical closeness; it's whether the two people are in the same spot concerning closeness. What may be sufficient for one couple may be excessively little for another. There's no best quality level except for on the off chance that one individual needs to kiss and snuggle constantly and the other is, in reality, somewhat bashful or awkward with closeness, then there is probably going to be a jumble. So, if you like the sum, at that point, it's all acceptable! On the off chance that you don't, at that point, something isn't adjusting for you, and you should converse with your spouse to see where they are at."

Advantages of Physical Intimacy

1. It's a statement of adoration

Probably the main motivation why physical closeness is significant in a love story is because this is one of the premier manners by which spouses express their adoration for each other. At the point when a love affair needs sexual science and actual fondness, it is bound to fizzle. This intimate time you spend together is passionate, exciting, and delivers oxytocin and dopamine. This hormone and synapse are the results of feeling nearer to your mate, trust, satisfaction, and even habit. It's no a big surprise why physical closeness is so significant in love life.

2. Physical closeness decreases pressure

One of the advantages of sex is that it limits mental pressure and tension. Being genuinely close to your partner lowers pulse and diminish pressure reactions in your mind. Furthermore, it isn't simply sex. Different types of physical closeness, for example, embracing or hand-holding, can trigger the arrival of oxytocin. This hormone will, at that point, trigger the cerebrum's prize and delight focuses, which brings down the passion of nervousness. One examination had members routinely captivating in intercourse for about fourteen days to see its impact on pressure and uneasiness. The outcomes uncovered cell development in the hippocampus, which is the very region of the cerebrum that manages pressure.

3. Closeness with mate assembles trust

Consistently, trust is worked after some time when a few becomes more acquainted with each other's actual steadfastness, examples, and conduct. In any case, in the heart, or should we say mind, trust is frequently set off by the arrival of oxytocin. Trust is an enormous piece of connections. At the point when two individuals trust each other, they feel more liberated to act naturally, aren't dubious of an outsider entering the love story, and can be more open, genuine, and open to their companion. This is one of the advantages of sex as well. While having intercourse or nestling close on the sofa, the cerebrum discharges oxytocin, a hormone that makes individuals additionally trusting and open to social cooperation.

4. Improved closeness outside the room

The closer you are in the room, the more associated you will feel outside of it. There is an extraordinary significance of touch in a relationship, and it remains constant in any event for nonsexual closeness.

Being actually close with your companion is probably the greatest way you, in a real sense, associate. Nonsexual demonstrations of closeness, like clasping hands, nestling, strolling arm constantly, and being all the more genuinely lively are some caring articulations that come after sex. Since closeness raises levels of adoration boosting oxytocin and vasopressin, it's nothing unexpected that couples who consistently engage in sexual relations become more friendly with each other in different parts of life.

5. Physical closeness helps your immunity

There are advantages of sex, both intellectually and genuinely. Getting physically involved with your mate can directly affect your invulnerable framework. The resistant framework gets a lift during sexual excitement and climax.

At the point when you are routinely explicitly dynamic with your spouse, you will bring the antibodies up in your framework that are answerable for battling against infections and germs that make you weak.

6.   Physical closeness raises the spirit

Another significance of the actual romance is that sex can support the spirit. One investigation even puts a financial incentive on it, recommending that couples who have intercourse once seven days increase a greater resolve help than they would if they acquired an extra $50,000 every year. Since physical closeness in a love affair supports dopamine, it causes you to feel more joyful. Climax aside, one Swedish investigation proposes that the love precedes and after sex that offers a lift in confidence.

7.   It advances science

They are actually private methods of engaging in sexual relations with each other and sharing individual snapshots of closeness. These can go from a sweet touch, a waiting kiss on the lips, or interesting vicinity. This conduct advances science and sexual expectation. This desire carries fervor to the love life and causes couples to feel more associated.

8.   Medical advantages

Numerous medical advantages come from being actually close with your spouse. For instance, having intercourse routinely can bring down a man's danger of creating prostate cancer growth. Being truly cozy without sex additionally has its advantages. Couples rest better and feel more like each other when they snuggle in bed. Oxytocin delivered by actual contacting and sex can likewise soothe torment and migraines, help you decompress, and lessen numerous types of actual ailment.

9. Causes you to look and to feel more youthful

There might be a connection between's a truly personal relationship and how youthful you look. The estrogen and testosterone delivered during sex might be giving your body an energetic, solid gleam.

10. Expands romance fulfillment

Contact is a solid sensation, both truly and inwardly. It raises passion for security, comfort, love, perkiness, sensation, and the sky is the limit from there. Couples who are genuinely close report a higher pace of romantic fulfillment. At the point when mates draw in each other with actual contacting, sexual or else, it causes them to feel thought about.

Other Forms of Intimacy

In each romance, closeness is critical. It is the thing that keeps the passionate flash alive for you and your spouse and furthermore keeps up a solid romance. In any case, frequently, we misjudge closeness for something more physical and disregard all different parts of a personal connection. While physical closeness is significant, there are different sorts of affections that are more critical and principal in a love story. A relationship between two individuals can't be estimated uniquely as far as physical closeness, as that may blur away with time. In any case, components like trust, similarity, and emotional partiality can construct and develop over the long run. This is just conceivable if different types of affections are likewise investigated.

Religious Closeness

Religious closeness reinforces a love affair and enables a couple to deal with life's emergencies obviously better than the ones who have not associated at this profound and existential level. Have you imparted your conviction about God to your better half? A few people accept that we cut our own fate while others accept that there is a more powerful that controls the course of our lives.

Where are you two on this? Is it safe to say that you are the two adherents? Do you have normal religious convictions? If not, this can put you and your spouse in extremely disparate ways throughout everyday life. For example, in case you're a skeptic or nonbeliever, and your mate is a devotee, it can prompt a ton of contrasts in your viewpoint and approach toward life circumstances.

It is essential to know where you both substitute connection to profound convictions and locate a shared opinion to work from, regardless of whether your perspectives don't correspond. It might likewise permit you to like each other's interpretation of life more and help cut back the distinctions and quarrels. On the off chance that your unique religious convictions don't coordinate, attempt to investigate new roads where you can tackle profound closeness as a team.

Tips to improve religious closeness

- Talk openly about your profound and strict convictions with your spouse.
- Try to pray, think, practice profound breathing, or sitting peacefully together.
- You can design a profound retreat or an escape that permits you to associate with nature to start your common religious excursion.
- Practice being present for at any rate 5 minutes, consistently when both of you center around one another and tune in to the sounds around you.
- Cleanse yourself from past experience, forgive, and let go.

Rational Closeness

Rational closeness is tied in with sharing thoughts and musings, aptitudes, side interests, and associating with one another on a cerebral level. Free-streaming conversations about what you pine for throughout everyday life, your viewpoint of various circumstances, the causes you feel firmly about, political belief systems, and ways of thinking are basic components of this kind of closeness. At the point when a couple is mentally close, they can discuss and contend, share, and comprehend unique perspectives without thinking about these distinctions literally. They additionally center around improving each other's rational capacities and supporting a spouse's development. It is tied in with understanding the idea of regard opposite one another's rational interests and perspectives. Rational closeness permits you to share everyone's disposition and conduct, offer productive analysis, but then make enough space in the love life to permit singular development. When a couple is mentally close, the two of them can examine significant parts of the romance, for example, how to bring up kids and oversee funds in a much more clear and compelling way.

Rational closeness is tied in with sharing thoughts and contemplations,

Tips to improve rational closeness

- Inculcate the propensity for perusing along with one another.
- Discuss your number one type of music, tunes, and verses with your mate.
- Make plans to do things together and team up on executing the arrangement. This will help improve your comprehension of how the other's brain works.
- Indulge in conversations about cultural development, ethical quality, craftsmanship, lifeways of thinking.
- Be each other's sounding board for significant life choices.
- Recognize and talk about how you can both develop as people and as a team.

Experiential Closeness

At the point when we talk about various sorts of closeness, the experiential measurement is maybe the least examined. Basically, it is tied in with gathering encounters altogether. While it is neither fitting nor feasible for any couple to hobnob, you should organize booking an ideal opportunity to do things together.

Be it week-by-week date evenings, going out at the ends of the week, going on outings, or doing things together around the house, these encounters assist you with making recollections that fortify your bond. Experiential closeness is tied in with interfacing with one another through shared encounters.

Tips to improve experiential closeness

- Create a rundown of things that you can do together and independently. The rundowns will help keep up a harmony between your own and shared space.
- Try to discover things that you both partake in and do them together. For instance, if you and your spouse appreciate exploring different avenues regarding food, cooking together can be an extraordinary method to develop experiential closeness.
- Take a stroll with your spouse, watch a film together or take a stab at planting as a team.
- Try to seek another leisure activity together. It very well may be anything from moving to ceramics, climbing, journey, or anything else that you both extravagant.
- Working out together is another incredible method to develop experiential closeness in your love story.

Dispute Closeness

At the point when two individuals meet up to share their life venture, it is difficult to maintain a strategic distance from clashes. This is the place where dispute closeness comes to play. This kind of closeness is about a couple's capacity to work their path contradictions in a socialized and aware way.

Compromise can be tied in with discovering shared belief to determine your disparities or essentially settling on a truce, or even a blend of the two, contingent upon the current circumstance.

While most couples figure out how to settle battles, do they truly resolve their disparities? Are there times when you accept you've figured out a contention, yet keep on encountering negative emotional buildup from it? Does an old issue keep coming up as an aggravation over and over?

Settling contentions and battles by brushing your issues away from plain view prompts hatred in the love affair. The focal point of this kind of closeness is to outfit a couple with the capacity to determine clashes reasonably. Whenever that is accomplished, your romance can climate the most unpleasant tempests and be more grounded for it.

Tips to improve dispute closeness

- You must stand by out the increased enthusiastic stage before your endeavor compromises. Examine your issues with a quiet psyche.
- Learn to impart your contemplations and insights openly with your mate. While you should be firm in passing on your viewpoint, don't be forceful.
- Respect your spouse in any event during the most unstable and troublesome periods of your romance.
- Change the outlook that arguments and battles are terrible for marriage. Acknowledge the way that arguments and contrast are a piece of a romance. How a couple haggles through these muddled stages is the thing that characterizes your quality as a couple.

Innovative Closeness

Innovative closeness implies searching for inventive approaches to help each other to remember the adoration, fondness, and bond that you share. This adorable part of causing each other to feel cherished and acknowledged frequently gets disregarded as a romance advances. That is the reason you hear endless couples complain that the passion is gone from their life.

Put your inventive cap on and find better approaches to amaze your mate together with your demeanor of adoration.

Among all the various sorts of closeness, the inventive angle can have a gigantic effect and rapidly add more flavor to your romance. Regardless of how long you have been together, discover approaches to impractically play with your companion. Consider them and appreciate it when they give back.

Tips to improve inventive closeness

- Hand-composed notes about the things you acknowledge about your lifemate are an example that seldom disappoints. Hide these at key spots like their office pack or wardrobe, so they can risk upon them and be astonished.
- Write letters to one another.
- Send blossoms just because.
- Pamper them with the correct blessings occasionally.
- Plan passionate date evenings frequently.

How To Increase Intimacy

What rates are most elevated in a drawn-out romance? Enthusiasm is significant, positively, yet closeness rates are most elevated. That is the thing that was found in the analysis of Robert J. Sternberg in a review of conjugal fulfillment among 101 grown-ups who'd been together for as meager as a year and up to 42 years.

Closeness is the feeling of someone else completely knowing you and cherishing you given what your identity is — just as disregarding it. This requires bringing a jump into uncommon trustworthiness and permitting yourself to be defenseless. The more profound the closeness, the more you'll have the experience of all-out retention with your spouse, all through the bed. For a few, closeness is that feeling of being "home" within sight of your mate. Or on the other hand, it very well might be an expanded feeling of loosened-up delight when you see your cherished one's face after nonattendance.

Closeness is the way into a cheerful and sound long-haul romance. Love life closeness requires a solid physical and passionate association. At the point when a love story needs closeness, it very well may be hard to keep up. If a degree of association is inadequate with regards to it, it can prompt passion of dejection and hatred. At the point when you feel sincerely cozy with your mate, it builds your general prosperity. If you notice the close association with your spouse isn't what you need it to be, read on for 10 different ways to expand the degree of closeness in your love affair.

1. Take a stab at Something New

An everyday schedule can assist you with having a sense of security. You realize what's in store and what will occur straightaway. In a love life, this can give a degree of security. Nonetheless, taking a stab at something new and surprises can help reignite the sparkle that can keep your love story fascinating. Venturing out of your customary range of familiarity and taking a stab at something new can be animating. It doesn't generally make a difference what it is that you do. You can pick up something together, attempt an action that is new to both of you, or take a stab at something in the room you haven't attempted previously. At the point when you explore new territory and distinctive together, the energy produced by the experience can make incitement and association that can assist you with feeling nearer to one another.

2. Think back

Think back about the great occasions you've shared together. At the point when you examine a pleasant encounter you had together or something entertaining you saw, it transports you back to that time as you review the feelings encompassing the occasion. At the point when you think back about pleasurable encounters you had, you recover a portion of the good passion identified with those encounters. On the off chance that you are attempting to expand your couple's closeness, you need to zero in on the great recollections and what they resembled at that point. Thinking back about the positive encounters helps maintain the emphasis on what is going right in your love affair, which can develop your couple's closeness.

3. Touch Eachother More

Actual contact causes you to remain associated with your spouse. Contact is the first of the faculties to create and is a basic segment of sound turn of events. Warm and actual touch has various medical advantages too. The medical advantages incorporate a diminishing for the pulse and an expansion in the holding hormone, oxytocin. This happens for the individual being contacted just like the one doing the contacting. So, connect and touch your mate. Clasp hands when going for a stroll, stroke their leg while sitting together, and wait when you give them an embrace. Invest more energy contacting each other to build your degree of closeness.

4. Set a Timetable for Sex

Focus on sex once more. As unromantic as it would appear, life can impede your sexual association if it's not on the timetable. At the point when you slither into bed following a monotonous day, at times, the main thing at the forefront of your thoughts is rest. It is simpler to abandon sex when you're not prone to do it. Notwithstanding, on the off chance that it is essential for the planned daily schedule, the private association that you get through sexual closeness will stay a significant piece of your love life. Booked sex gives the occasion to construct the expectation and connect with the greatest erogenous zone, the mind. You can send instant messages paving the way to the sex date depicting what you need to do and how attractive you find your spouse. It additionally allows you to plan for alone time where the emphasis can be on one another. At the point when you participate in consistently arranged sexual closeness, you are bound to be available to more unconstrained sexual experiences also.

5. Remain Connected

Remain in touch with your spouse for the duration of the day. Text one another, leave little notes for your mate and let them realize how your day is going. Check in with one another once per day and inspect each other's eyes. See how your spouse goes through their day and offer your encounters too. Get to know each other in the nights. Examine things other than the children, tasks, and timetables. At the point when you feel a solid connection with your spouse, your degree of closeness will improve.

6. Show Appreciation

Saying please and thank you can go far towards helping your mate feel increased in value. At the point when you feel that your spouse acknowledges you, it is simpler to do the everyday tasks that help your family unit run all the more easily. Be explicit and earnest with your commendation. Praise your spouse unreservedly. Tell them what you love about them. Basic thoughtful gestures and expressions of commendation can help you both feel more esteemed by the other. Feeling that your mate acknowledges you reinforcing your couple's bond.

7. Go On A Date

Go out on the town outside of your home with your spouse. Create an opportunity to be with your spouse in an alternate climate where the emphasis can be on one another. At the point when you are at home, there can be a ton of interruptions from children, work, or errands. Without the entirety of the external impedance, you can zero in on partaking in one another and having a great time together. Going on dates together helps maintain the attention on your association as a team.

8. Be Vulnerable

You should be open to your mate to feel acknowledged and comprehended. Being defenseless can be awkward, particularly from the outset. Offer your emotions, your concerns, your apprehensions, your energy, your interests, and your fantasies with your spouse. Put forth an attempt to have those awkward discussions that you regularly attempt to stay away from. Tell your spouse when you are feeling harmed or unreliable in your love story. Your closeness with your mate will increment when you trust you can be open to your spouse.

9. Have A Life Outside Of Your Love affair

Even though your love life should be a need, on the off chance that you need to expand your closeness, respecting your individual necessities will make you a superior spouse. At the point when you deny your necessities or depend just on your mate to satisfy them, you are setting your romance up for disappointment. On the off chance that you are satisfied in different aspects of your life, you will have more to provide for your love story. Invest energy with companions and take part in diversions and exercises that you feel enthusiastic about. At the point when you have something in your life that energizes and feeds you outside of your love affair, you can impart your excitement to your spouse, which can assist you with developing nearer.

10. Backing Your Spouse

Be there for your spouse when they need you. If they approach you for help, told them what you may or may not be able to help. Tell them that you are there. Be a decent audience. Utilize fundamental social abilities and rehash back what you hear them state, so they feel heard. Put down your telephone, limit different interruptions and give your mate your full focus. Cheer your spouse on and be trustworthy. At the point when your spouse feels like you are there for them and they can rely on you, it can reinforce your couple association.

A solid couple association exists when emotional and physical closeness is a need. If the above tips are not viable, or if other social issues meddle with closeness, couples advising can help. Improving your love life closeness is justified, despite all the trouble, as it can improve your association and your general individual prosperity also.

11. Relish In Your Solace and Association.

At the point when we are first beginning dating somebody, everything is new and energizing. We experience extraordinary feelings as we become acquainted with the individual and become intimate with one another. After some time, however, this curiosity and energy reduction. While this can be frustrating, there is a flip side: the association is more profound than at any other time, connoted by the solace you feel in one another's organization. In this way, you can improve your closeness with your mate by recollecting the underlying phases of your love story, valuing its turn of events, and savoring exactly how agreeable you feel with your companion.

12. Switch Up Your Daily Schedule.

Then again, it's likewise useful to switch up your schedule once in a while to instigate those serious feelings once more. Make a special effort to do the unforeseen and astonish your companion. For instance, book an end-of-the-week escape and have all that all set — book the inn, gather the sacks, top the vehicle off with gas. You can likewise switch up your everyday practice and improve closeness by parting ways. There's nothing amiss with going on isolated outings sometimes. This will allow you to miss one another, and you'll feel upbeat and energized when you're brought together.

13. Keep Up Great Roads of Correspondence.

Frequently, we don't put aside an ideal opportunity to have an appropriate discussion with our companion — be it about the adoration we have for them or, then again, an issue in the love affair. Nonetheless, keeping up great roads of correspondence can enhance our work to improve closeness and keep that fire alive. Connections are steady work and can self-destruct if there isn't exertion placed in to look after it. Little things go far while looking after closeness, and hatred can rapidly develop if there are bad roads of correspondence. Knowing and disclosing to your mate consistently why you're infatuated with them and how you feel about them is another approach to keep the fire copying. Differing is likewise a significant part of any love life. Having the option to serenely and deferentially tell your spouse issues you're having is basic for looking after closeness. "Quietness is the quiet enemy of connections."

14. Exhibit Your Affection Frequently.

Make a propensity out of indicating to your mate that you love, care for, and uphold them. A large number of us expect or demand that our spouses realize we love them — yet that doesn't mean we shouldn't remind our lifemates through both our words and our activities consistently. For instance, when your companion returns home from work, inspect their eyes and afterward kiss them. Ask how their day was. Put gas in their vehicle. Compose an adorable directive for them to discover on the whiteboard in the kitchen. Discover little approaches to advise them that you give it a second thought. This will assist with improving your life mate and keep that fire-consuming inconclusively.

15. Reveal More to Feel Nearer.

Over the long haul, without proceeding with mindfulness, it is anything but difficult to lose that inclination to continue finding everything to think around each other. People that therapists have named openers have intimate discussions with others since something about them encourages revelation. The individuals who don't open up or make it simple for others to do as such, known as high self-screens, have a more troublesome time with intimate connections.

16. Set Aside a Few Minutes for Profoundly Emotional Discussions.

These are among the occasions individuals feel nearest. At the point when we share our musings toward the day's end when we're sufficiently fortunate to have the option to do that, it feels cozy.

17. Experiment Together.

One lady shared occasions where she and her spouse feel nearest, including when they have a beneficial discussion about something whereupon they oppose this idea. Yet in addition, she let me know, "is the point at which we produce something together. 'Raising' of the felines, accomplishing something truly decent for companions or family. Like when we're in a state of harmony about 'we should do such-and-such for someone or other.'"

18. Relish the Daily Practice.

At the point when we're different from each other, whatever we learn is unforeseen, bringing about exceptional feelings. Slowly over the long run, we become more unsurprising to each other. However, there's a positive side to this consistency. It prompts closeness, in which the spouses are so associated with one another that the one doesn't perceive the other is there, similarly as the air we inhale can be underestimated, notwithstanding its need to live.

19. Guarantee That It's Protected to Be Open.

Imagine a scenario in which you are essential for a befuddled couple, where you long for a more profound degree of informative transparency than your mate actually will. Solace levels with verbal sharing regularly increment with training in a genuinely protected setting, so keep on working at turning into a non-critical audience.

20. Consider Whether You're a Superior Match Than You Might Suspect.

Individuals differ concerning how much closeness they need to maintain a strategic distance from depression and the amount they can endure before feeling immersed. Those with more grounded needs will work more enthusiastically to guarantee cozy contact with their spouses by listening all the more intently and asking their spouses to be more expressive. On the off chance that the need is more vulnerable, at that point, there will be a more fragile connection between closeness and love story fulfillment. As such, on the off chance that you don't want the degree of absolute closeness I'm discussing here, you presumably wouldn't fret if your spouse isn't that excited about sharing their own internal life, all things considered.

21. Closeness Is More Than Words or Sex.

Just 33% of the separated men in the example above said they didn't locate the passionate closeness they needed. What some of them missed, however, was their spouses being there for them "in a lot more full ways." They needed solid exhibitions of closeness, for example, being kissed or asked how they are toward the day's end and being welcomed with great enthusiasm at the entryway. However, the less well-spoken exhibit their affection in their own particular manners, they merit credit for their insightful conduct, just as additional persistence and comprehension concerning the discussion denied.

22. Constantly Share Your Cravings.

Over the long haul, enthusiasm blurs. Anticipate it, and hope to work on the off chance that you need to keep things hot. At the point when you feel the fire beginning to wear out, take control and speak with your mate. In case you're exhausted, odds are they are, as well. The best way to make it work is to do it together.

23. Send a Sext.

Rather than 'what's for supper?' take a stab at adding some sex to your writings by communicating something specific about what you need to do when they return home. Try not to be hesitant to get explicit. Review insights concerning perhaps the most smoking experience, depict an outfit you'll be wearing — or possibly send a pic of yourself in it. An unforeseen hot message to your spouse is an extraordinary method to assemble that pressure for the duration of the day, so when they return home, you both know it's go time.

24. Watch Pornography Together.

Pornography shouldn't be something you mind your own business. Take a stab at discovering something you both like. It'll get you in the temperament and give a few thoughts for pretending or places that you'd prefer to attempt. If pornography isn't your thing, take a stab at playing a provocative game utilizing sensual writing. Locate a sensual story or novel and alternate perusing to one another. Perceive the number of pages you can traverse before you can't remain quiet about your hands.

25. Make Your Own Erotica.

Get a diary to pass among you. One individual beginning the suggestive story, and the other gets back on track. On the off chance that you need to make it truly unstable, consent to no sex for seven days while you're composing your hot story. Before the week's over, you will blast to get your hands on each other.

26. Send Your Spouse a "Unique Conveyance."

While preparing toward the beginning of the day, ensure your mate observes you putting on underwear. At that point, as the day goes on, send a surprise by dropping off the undergarments in an envelope at their office.

27. Make a Sexual Container List.

In case you're in a romance, the odds are acceptable that one of you has referenced an imagination or two. It's an ideal opportunity to make a portion of those a reality. Next time you're out to supper or hanging out at home, set out the test to record five things you'd each need to attempt explicitly. At that point, trade records, see what you shared for all intents and purpose, and pick a few things you're both ready to attempt.

28. Switch Your Contraception.

Consult your gynecologist or obstetrician before thinking about this choice. I didn't understand how low my longing had gotten until after I quit utilizing the Pill. While this won't work for everybody, it did wonders for some.

29. Shop for Sex Toys Together.

Simply the action of setting off to a sex-toy store and looking for them together could be a great behavior for a couple to attempt.

30. Establish the Ideal Sexual Climate for Yourself.

Making the correct setting for the most private, energizing, and satisfying sex for her was the way to spicing up her sexual coexistence. Thinking about past sexual encounters that were quite pleasurable has shown me what works and what doesn't. For instance, I have the best sex when my pressure is low, after a long, sumptuous back massage, and when I'm feeling in adoration with my body — to give some examples of things.

31. Attempt Masturbation Together.

It is so damn hot to observe each other masturbate; in addition to it requires some investment than different types of spouse sex.

32. See a Sex Advisor.

On the off chance that a sexual respite endures, sex treatment is consistently a possibility for you and your spouse to find further purposes for sexual issues and, thus, discover approaches to address them.

The Benefit For The Couple about The Knowledge Of Sexual Position

A sex position is a place of the body that individuals use for sex or other sexual exercises. Sexual acts are commonly depicted by the positions the members receive to play out those demonstrations. Although sex, in general, includes the entrance of the member of one individual by another, sex positions ordinarily include penetrative or non-penetrative sexual exercises.

Three classes of sex are usually polished: vaginal intercourse (including vaginal infiltration), anal entrance, and oral sex (particularly mouth-on-genital stimulation). Sex acts may likewise include different types of genital incitement; for example, solo or shared masturbation, which may include scouring or infiltration by the utilization of fingers or hands, or by a gadget (sex toy, for example, a dildo or vibrator). The demonstration may likewise include anilingus. There are various sex places that members may receive in any of these sorts of sex or acts; a few creators have contended that the quantity of sex positions is basically boundless.

Sex certainly has a lot of physical and mental advantages. In any case, the response to how significant it is in a marriage is a touch more confounded than that. Regular sexual behavior has advantages, for example, diminished pressure, emotional association, more noteworthy closeness, and brought down separation rates. There are contrasts in how people see sex, however, it assumes a vital part in marriage.

Why Sex Positions Are Important in a Marriage

1. Sex Positions Promotes Intimacy

This is presumably the most evident motivation behind why hitched couples need to have more sex. Sex assembles closeness. Indeed, you share everything, and there's a decent bond in your romance, but then if sex positions are low by the way you express your adoration for one another, something's wrong. Living respectively and the conviction of one another's quality can make your science burn out. Although you're in love, you may have lost the sexual science you had toward the start, so what you need is somewhat more sex to bring it back.

2. It Relieves from Stress

It's obviously how stunning it very well may be to get back home following a difficult day and deliver all that repressed pressure energy with your spouse in bed. Specialists state that ordinary sex encourages individuals to react better to pressure because of the arrival of feel-good endorphins in the body. In addition to the fact that it helps you unwind, yet it gives a lot of holding time with your mate in bed. And afterward, there's all the acceptable night's rest you'll get after that. Albeit a decent workout isn't suggested long before rest, sex is a special case for it. It is seen that it diminishes internal heat levels and advances profound rest.

3. Sex Positions Increases the Bonds Between Couples

The explosion of endorphins in the cerebrum after sexual behavior is liable for helping couples bond during sex. It isn't just about entrance and completing, yet the lively investigation that precedes it that will give you the most intimate minutes with your spouse. The two people need enthusiasm, passion, and science to show each other that their adoration is alive and progressing admirably.

4. Sex Positions helps in Problem-tackling

As time advances in an involved acquaintance, couples differ more on things than they did before toward the beginning of the romance. Clashes because of the distinction of feeling become typical, and couples will, in general, float separated. Sex at that point turns into an important behavior to make a ceasefire. Sexual closeness assists couples with working through their contradictions all the more affectionately as they look past their disparities to discover shared conviction that works for both as opposed to participating in a force battle. It additionally revives lost passion and helps them to remember the trust they share even in the center of their hardest battles.

5. Sex Positions Builds a Better Communication Level

Explicitly fulfilled couples will disclose to you that sex isn't limited distinctly to the room; its underlying foundations expand well past into their regular daily existences. Reciprocity outside your room is the key – without it, your actual association in the bed would be feeble. Extraordinary sex begins in the brain, which incorporates legitimate companionship with your spouse consistently. Developing to it is the thing that makes sex quite a lot more agreeable, particularly for ladies; it encourages them to feel a profound association with their man and really love the intercourse.

6. Sex Positions Are Great Exercises

Sex being the actual vivacious action that it is, causes you to consume many calories. A decent round of sex is equal to some direct action, for example, energetic strolling or climbing a stairway. You likewise assemble muscles during sex, which assist you with fixing and tone your mid-region, lower back, and thighs. Normally, you would wind up consuming 200 calories shortly after good sex. In this way, in case you're on a workout schedule observing all the calories you admission and consume, removing a brief period on the treadmill, and subbing it with sex with your spouse has exacerbated benefits.

7. Sex Positions Builds Better Self-regard

Sex is critical to feel extraordinary about yourself. No one appreciates being in a marriage that needs actual enthusiasm. Everyone needs to be wanted. Thusly, energetic and empowering sex is a pointer that your mate is still into you. Being incredible in bed and having your partner return to you needing more is an extraordinary confidence sponsor for the two people. Then again, analyzing how significant sex is in a drawn-out love affair shows that a flamed-out science or being shaky about yourself and performing inadequately can ultimately drive your spouse to search for different methods outside the marriage.

8. Sex Positions Have Numerous Physical Benefits

Not exclusively can sex give you decent exercise and consume calories, yet it likewise has various actual medical advantages for both you and your spouse. The muscles associated with sex are finely conditioned, improving bladder control in both of them. The endorphins delivered during sexual behavior help to ease actual painfulness and, in some cases, even headaches and back torment, improving serenity and prosperity. Sex with your mate is additionally a decent cardio workout alongside having a lot of advantages for the heart, for example, bringing down circulatory strain thereafter and diminishing odds of coronary illness.

CHAPTER 2:

Sex Positions

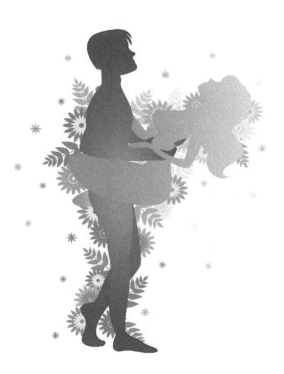

In life, it is best to leave some things on repeat, but your sex routine better not be one of those. Regardless of how hot the spark in the bedroom is, you still need brand new sex positions to rekindle the flames every now and then; else, things can get really boring.

Every time you come up in the bedroom with something new and fresh, you get yourself ready for a far more stimulating and fun experience and, of course, a bigger finish. The reality is that your brain looks for newness, and it takes part in the satisfaction and excitement, especially for women.

This can also be a wonderful idea for your love life. The most significant challenge that is there for intimacy is the loss of newness in the bedroom. Exploring on the sheets increases emotional intimacy while encouraging growth and risk-taking. Newer sex positions go a long way in encouraging you and your spouse to be more open with each other in the bedroom and everywhere else. And afterward, you'll discover that your love story has developed better trust.

At times, exchanging up positions may even be an unquestionable requirement. In case you're thinking 'ouch' when the proposal of sex is put on the table, you could profit by investigating different places that are more agreeable for people with assorted capacities, just as those with persistent torment, or painfulness from penetration. Yet, even whenever you've discovered that torment-free position, that doesn't mean it's your lone choice. While it's anything but difficult to turn into an animal of propensity when you've nailed that go-to, agreeable, peak each time position, Parks urges you to keep blending it up. There are numerous potential outcomes out there that your creative mind probably won't have even idea up yet.

Be that as it may, sex is fundamental for our psychological and actual wellbeing. Sex can improve our disposition, make us less focused, and encourage better rest. That is the reason — on the off chance that you can — you should continue having it! One approach to get you more amped up for having intercourse is to toss some assortment into your sexual coexistence by evaluating different sex positions.

New sex positions are something you and your spouse could feel free to test, well, at this moment, on the off chance that you both needed to. However, before we dive into less run of the mill sex positions (and minor departure from a portion of the old works of art like missionary, cowgirl, spooning, and doggy style), we need to pose you one inquiry: What are you planning to accomplish by switching up sex positions?

If your spouse has a vulva and you're searching for positions to help them climax, at that point, you need to search for sex positions where you can physically invigorate your mate's clitoris while penetrating them. Most ladies won't have the option to get profoundly stirred or have a climax except if there's some sort of clitoral incitement occurring.

Maybe you're searching for more mental excitement. At that point, possibly you need to evaluate a place that feels hasty. Provided that this is true, search for positions where you can push your spouse in a bad spot or engage in sexual relations on a hard surface.

On the other hand, perhaps you need to take a stab at something new for novelty. Simply note that these positions are not ideal from beginning to end. You will probably need to blend and match positions. You can begin with more gutsy and exceptionally athletic positions, yet then progress into a less requesting position where you can completely unwind and feel present in the sex you're having.

A portion of these positions won't feel unfathomable at the first run-through. They may take a couple of attempts to get the hang of it. What's more, some can conceivably be perilous — not in an attractive way, but rather in a painful way. Try not to try too hard. This isn't a "push through the torment" circumstance. If a position doesn't feel right, at that point, change to another.

Examples of Different Sex Position

1. **Advanced Cow:** For the classic Cow position, the woman stands with her feet separated while the man penetrates her from behind. Then, she bends over to touch the floor with her hands. Meanwhile, for this advanced version of the Cow position, the man would hold on to the woman's waist as she takes her feet off from the ground.

2. **Advanced Crab Walk:** Remember the crab walk you did in gym classes while in grammar school? Both of you and your mate will get into the crab walk position; then the woman lowers herself onto her mate's penis or the dildo. The woman can do two things. She can lift her hips up or down, or she may gyrate. She can do whatever feels better at any moment for her and her spouse.

3. **Advanced High Squeeze:** For the High Squeeze sex position, the female mate lies on her back and places her feet on the man's chest. Then, he can enter her while kneeling from under her feet. Even when this classic version of high squeeze can be very comfortable for women, the advanced version may not be as relaxing. For this variation, the man has to raise his knees up, and the female mate's hips are away from the ground; therefore, she will have to rest on her upper back.

4. **Aquarius:** If you find yourself really amazing with doing bridges, go for one. Then, your spouse can penetrate you. While they do this, make sure you wrap your legs around their butt. That means you're half-suspended now. They can definitely handle the thrusting from this position, but you too can always step in and serve as a power bottom. This way, you can, if you feel like, demonstrate your acrobatic ability.

5. **Ballet Dancer:** If you try Ballet Dancer standing up against the wall of a bedroom, in the shower, or the kitchen, the two spouses need to be supportive; they can lean on each other and embrace themselves throughout the way. While standing on one foot, turn towards your spouse and make the other leg wrapped around his waist as they help to support you.

6. **Belly Down:** Lay on your stomach with your hands in the middle of your legs. Then, grind your legs together by moving your hips up and then down continuously. Thusly, your clitoris and the erogenous zone around it will rub against your immovably held fingers.

7. **Bubble the Fun:** Let your body lowered and legs hanging out of a bathing tub; begin by surrendering yourself to a rubdown at the top before you descend to meander around in the water. Unwinding in a tub with warm, sweet-smelling water assuages tension, eases pressure, and certainly gets you feeling great.

8. **Butter Churner (Squat Thruster):** Lie down on your back and have your legs raised and collapsed over so that your lower legs are on one or your other sides, while the man squats and inserts their penis, finger, lash on, or dildo all through your vagina. Besides getting that eye-to-eye connection, the additional surge of blood that goes in your head will help to build delight. It gets a greater amount of your faculties included, amplifying up the whole experience.

9. **Champagne Room:** The male partner sits while the female sits on top, looking away. It makes it easy for her to direct the movement and force of the pushes. Have a go at doing it on the steps or the bathtub edge.

10. **Circle Perk:** While in a sitting position, move your finger in a circular manner encircling your clit as if you are drawing a circle with it. Start gradually and speed up the movement and pressure, contingent upon your response. This is a move that is incredible for ladies who see direct clitoral weight as excessively exceptional for delayed incitement.

11. **Classic Chair Sex Position:** One spouse sits in a seat with their feet placed on the floor. Then, the other spouse rides them, bringing down themselves onto the penis or dildo; the person straddling can put their hands on their mate's shoulders to keep them consistent while they get in position. At that point, clutching their shoulders, neck, the seat, or nothing by any means, move to different directions to discover what feels best.

12. **Closed for Business:** Some women find direct clitoral incitement awkward. Having their legs closed during oral stimulation may help. The man should have his hand over their erogenous zones while applying light weight; at that point, rub your tongue firmly on the region near the clitoris to add aberrant pleasure.

13. **Cockscrew:** Stay at the edge of a seat or bed. Lay on your hip and lower arm and bring your thighs pressed together. The male partner then stands and rides you, entering or pounding from behind. If you keep your legs squeezed together in this position, it will give your partner a tighter hang as they push. Rather than letting your man accomplish all the sweet work, take a stab at pushing your hips marginally to coordinate the beat.

14. **Couch Grind:** This position involves you riding on the arm of a stuffed seat or lounge chair or a table edge with a thick blanket or towel placed on top of it. Start with moving the hips a bit and gradually gather speed. This is extraordinary if you like strong, consistent tension on or around your clitoris.

15. **Couch Surfer (The Lazy Susan):** Convenient for fast sex and adds flavor outside the room. Request your spouse to twist her body over the arm from a lounge chair as you, the man, enters from behind. They can pound on the firm, however comfortable arm for various incitement with insignificant exertion.

16. **Cowboy:** The woman lies on her back while her spouse rides her. The man can, at that point, delicately embed their penis, lash on, or finger through the tight opening made by her semi-shut legs. The tightness builds the pleasure of penetration. The man can also stroke her bosoms or delicately hold down her wrists for a minimal servitude activity.

17.   **Cowgirl:** The woman stoops on top, pushing off her spouse's chest while sliding their thighs in all directions. You can soothe a portion of your weight from his pelvis by reclining and supporting yourself on his thighs. By being in control in this position, you'll be in total control of his and your orgasms. Find new sensations by broadening your knees and carrying them closer to his body.

18.   **Cowgirl Leaning Back (Cowgirl Astride):** This is a great sex position that originates from cowgirl. Jump on top as you would in Cowgirl; however, this time, rest your body in reverse with your hands propped on the man's knees. For extra help, they can clutch your buttocks. With this position, you'll get a great stimulation of the G-spot. This position accompanies the reward of simple admittance to the clitoris.

19.   **Cowgirl's Helper (Cowgirl with a Forward Bend):** Fold forward while in the cowgirl position for extraordinary G-spot stimulation. Instead of skipping all over, lay your body on top of your mate's while kissing and caressing their body. You could even pull his hair.

20.   **Cross Your Heart:** This position requires that the lady lies back and places her feet on her mate's chest. He bows and enters her from under the legs. The lady may fold her legs at the lower legs. The strain brought about by her crossed legs will make practically any movement pleasurable, so have some good times investigating.

21.   **Cross-Booty:** The man enters as in the missionary position; at that point, shifts their chest and legs away from your body so that his pelvis is in a similar area; however, their appendages create an "X" with yours. You feel a greater amount of your spouse's body moving with this sex position. Utilize this extraordinary point to rub their back, butt, or legs as they push. Both of you will go insane from enjoying this position.

22. **David Copperfield (Trick and Treat):** Place a cushion under their hips to tilt their pelvis up. Curve their knees so they can put their feet on your shoulder bones.

23. **Doggy Style (Man's Best Friend):** This could be your best course of action in the wake of beginning with The Flatiron position. Entering your mate from behind, you'll have the option to push profound so the tip of your penis contacts their cervix, a regularly ignored delight zone. In any case, you ought to do this gradually and delicately. A few women think that it's difficult.

24. **Face-Off (The Lap Dance):** Sit on a seat or the edge of the bed. Your spouse, at that point, faces you, folds their arms over your back, jumps on top, and sits on your lap. Once in the seat, they can ride here and there on your penis by squeezing with their legs or knees. Need to speed up? Help by getting their posterior and lifting and skipping.

25. **Fire and Ice:** Head to the shower and let the warm water run everywhere on your spouse's body. At that point, dissolve ice in your mouth before giving them oral. The combo of your cool mouth and the high temp water running everywhere on their body will be awesome, and an extraordinary transition into astounding shower sex.

26. **Fitness Friends:** You lie on your side with one of your legs lifted, and your spouse sits on their knees, rides your base leg, and penetrates you while adjusting your lower leg on their shoulder.

27. **Flatiron (Downward Dog, The Belly Flop):** Lie face down on the bed, legs straight, hips somewhat raised. This sex position makes a cozy fit, so your mate's penis or lash-on will appear to be much bigger. For comfort and to expand the point of their hips, they can put a pad under their lower abs.

You enter them from behind and keep your weight off their body by propping yourself up with your arms. Some shallow pushes and profound breathing will enable the frolic to last more.

28. **Froggy-Style (Jump Frog):** In this variety of doggy styles, you'll prop your head on your lower arms and your lower arms on the bed (as opposed to remaining in a table-top position). As in doggy style, this position makes it simple for you to contact yourself while your spouse pushes.

29. **Get to the G-Spot:** Let the woman lie on her back with her knees pressed against her chest. Input a couple of fingers profoundly into her vagina. As you pull out your finger, press against the front of your vagina and urethra and twist your finger in an alluring signal.

30. **Gift Wrapped (The Horny Mantis):** Relaxing situation with more profound entrance and expanded closeness. Both of you lie on your sides, confronting each other. Your spouse curves and spreads their legs and points their vagina toward you. You lift your legs between theirs to enter while they fold their legs over your back.

31. **Golden Arch:** Your spouse sits with their legs straight and you sit on top of them with bowed knees on top of their thighs, and you both recline. This position gives you both decent perspectives on one another's full bodies. You'll additionally have command over the profundity, speed, and point of the pushes. They can utilize their hand to rub your clitoris or use yours. Recline farther for additional G-spot incitement.

32. **H2Ohh Yeah (Aquaman's Delight):** A form of The Ballet Dancer position. Your mate's lightness in the water makes this sex position simpler to hold. And you should simply move some swimsuit material far removed of certain body parts; the lifeguards will be unaware.

33. **Heir to the Throne (Lazy Girl):** Let your spouse sit on a seat with their legs fully open. You take it from that point. This is a decent sex position for either starting the moderate development with free, wide strokes or finishing with solid pull. Your spouse can, without much of a stretch, guide you, and they're ready to get a full perspective on you between her legs, which is a turn-on for some individuals.

34. **Hovering Butterfly (The Face Sitter):** They can coordinate the situation of your tongue and the weight against them by ascending or pushing down. Your mate rides you setting their knees at your ears. They can clutch a headboard or wall for help. While you're doing your thing, they can use their fingers to brush their nipples or rub the highest point of their vulva.

35. **Iron Chef (Kitchen Confidential):** A variety of The Ballet Dancers in which your spouse raises their legs and folds them over your thighs or butt. Your kitchen counter is the ideal tallness for this tidbit.

36. **Kneeling Reach-Around:** While the individual with the vulva is in the doggy style position (as in on all fours, as their spouse penetrates from behind), the mate additionally stretches around to invigorate the clitoris. They can do this with either a toy or their hand.

37. **Leapfrog:** This is an altered doggy style. Jump on all fours, at that point, keeping hips raised, rest your head and arms on the bed. This sex position makes further penetrates — and allows you to lay on a cushion. Utilize your hands to stimulate your clitoris.

38. **Legs on the floor:** In this variation of the Missionary position, you'll lie on the bed with your legs hanging off. Put a cushion under your butt to keep your pelvis high. At that point, let your spouse remain at the end of the bed and lift your legs — you can fold them over his abdomen or spot them on his shoulders.

39. **Legs Up Missionary:** Starting in missionary position, the individual with the vulva rolls their hips back a piece so their legs are noticeable all around. From here, the male partner or mate with the dildo enters them while the woman lays their legs on their mate's shoulders.

40. **Look and Learn:** Hold a mirror, sit comfortably with one leg propped up on the bed or lounge chair. Since you can look at the merchandise, adventure away from your delicate clitoris to find new erogenous zones. Investigate the opening, inside, and back mass of your vagina with your fingers, squeezing and changing weight until you discover something that feels right.

41. **Magic Mountain:** Your spouse sits, legs bowed, reclining on all fours. You do likewise and afterward, creep toward them until you connect. You'll both feel truly associated taking a gander at one another. Increment your incitement by pounding your clitoris against their pelvis. Slide ice shapes down their chest and lets the cold water gather at the base of their pelvis.

42. **Missionary (The Matrimonial, Male Dominant):** Lots of eye and body contact. Lie on your back while they lie face down on top of you. This sex position is basic, rich, viable, and shockingly adaptable. Common, sure, however scrumptious. The most ordinarily utilized position on the planet, this is a particularly cozy position, taking into consideration vis-à-vis contact. You like it since you can control entrance profundity and speed of pushing. Your spouse appreciates feeling your weight on their body and the greatest skin-to-skin contact. Note that this position can make it harder to hold off discharge on account of the extraordinary stimulation and profound pushing. To protract lovemaking, start there, then change to a place that keeps up clitoral weight without such a great amount of pelvic to and fro.

43. **Missionary with A Pillow:** First, the individual with the vulva lays on the back with a cushion under their hips. At that point, the mate with the penis or dildo gets between their legs and enters them from above, as it were, with the two bodies corresponding to one another. It bodes well once you get into position. Guarantee.

44. **Modified Doggy Style:** Basically, you're getting into exemplary doggy style for this one, yet you're letting yourselves down, so you're either level on the bed with the penis or dildo proprietor on top, or the individual with the vulva can prop the two spouses up a piece by utilizing their elbows. This is really an incredible situation for individuals who love doggy style, however, have powerless wrists.

45. **Mountain Climber (The Pushup):** This position creates an extraordinary eye-to-eye connection, and it keeps the man's weight off her body. There's an explanation why people faint when they see a six-pack. They know a man with solid abs will be extraordinary in the sack. This position flaunts your quality and hard abs (on the off chance that you have them).

46. **Mutual Masturbation:** If you've dominated the craft of getting yourself off, at that point, this position is a simple one to do. Common masturbation is just about both, you and your spouse, jerking off simultaneously.

47. **Naughty Tee:** To handle another letter of the letter set, have your spouse lie on their side, confronting the highest point of the bed. Next, rests opposite to them, and hurry your hips down to meet theirs, twisting your knees and setting your feet level on the bed behind your mate's butt. Together, your bodies structure a T shape on the bed. From this position, your spouse can push into you.

48. **Olympus:** The way that the Olympus looks simple is a demonstration of how totally requesting different situations on this rundown are. Fold your legs over your spouse and have them hold you up — no dividers to incline toward. To make things extra testing, just hang on with one arm — let the other meander where it might.

49. **One Up (Over Your Shoulder, The Hamstring Stretch):** Kneel on the floor with your mate lying on the edge of the bed. Raise one of their legs and request that they uphold it by folding their hands over their hamstring just underneath the knee. With one hip raised, your mate will have the option to add some development to help in your stroking or to help move you to the ideal spot.

50. **Pirate's Bounty:** If the name isn't luring enough, this position is acceptable for profound addition and all-out clitoral incitement during intercourse. To play out Pirate's Bounty, the lady lays on her back with one leg on her mate's shoulder and the other folded over his thigh. The man is bowing. A cushion under the lady's back may make this position more agreeable.

51. **Post Position (Thighmaster):** Lie on your back and curve one of your legs, keeping the other outstretched. Your spouse rides the raised leg with a thigh on one or the other side and brings down themselves onto your part so their back is confronting you. They should hold your knee and use it for help as they rock here and there.

52. **Pushing' the Cushion:** This pleasant sex position requires a lounge chair and a vibrator. Accept an exemplary doggy-style position on the sofa, with the getting spouse confronting the rear of the lounge chair. Spot a cushion against your vagina, and spot a vibrator behind the pad. The vibrator will make the entire cushion shake and stimulate your clitoris while your mate enters you from behind. Sounds great, no?

53. **Quicker Picker Upper (The Pillow Driver):** A tad of assortment if missionary starts to feel flat; great chest area work out. Spot a cushion under the little of their back or their bum to tilt their pelvis and change the point of your entrance for various sensations. Preparing yourself with your hands on the bed as in a pushup position, you drop your weight from their body.

54. **Quickie Fix (The Bends):** Greater pushing force, and useful for fast in and out sex in your kitchen, particularly if your spouse is wearing a skirt. Request that they twist at the midriff and lay their hands on a household item, their knees, or the floor for help. You enter them from behind and hold their hips for help as you push.

55. **Restroom Attendant (Drop the Soap):** Slip into a restroom and request that they check the mirror while you enter them from behind. It lets you have an eye-to-eye connection during the G-spot-focusing on the back passage sex position.

56. **Reverse Cowgirl (Rodeo Drive, Half Way Around the World):** Lie on your back with your legs outstretched. Your spouse stoops close to you; at that point, turns and spreads their legs, riding your hips and confronting your feet. Bowing, your spouse drops down onto your penis and starts riding you.

57. **Reverse Scoop:** Get into the position of missionary, without separating, turn together onto your sides, utilizing your arms to help your chest areas. You get a similar full-body press and can look into one another's eyes. Take a stab at interlacing your legs with his or petting them down underneath.

58. **Scoop Me Up:** Both of you lie on your sides, confronting a similar heading. You bring your knees up somewhat while your spouse slides up behind your pelvis and enters you from behind. (You may likewise realize this as spooning.) This sex position considers more skin-to-skin contact, expanding your excitement. Let your mate place their hands on your shoulders to build the force and profundity of the push.

59. **Seated Oral:** First, you and your spouse need to pick who will get and who will be giving. Next, the collector sits in the seat and spreads their legs apart, while their spouse gives them orally.

60. **Seated Wheelbarrow:** This is similar, but it requires lesser energy. In this position, let your mate sit on the edge of the bed or sofa. You will go downward and afterward fold your legs over their abdomen, yet it's route simpler since you can rest your lower body on the bed instead of supporting your full weight.

61. **Seated Wrap-Around (the Seated Hug, Lotus Blossom):** This position requires you and your spouse to grasp one another—ideal for impractically looking into one another's eyes. One mate rides the other spouse while you both sit with folded legs.

The top mate folds their legs over the base spouse as you face one another and embrace. The base spouse enters the top mate vaginally with a toy or penis.

62. **Side by Side:** Lie on your side, confronting your spouse. At that point, lift your leg over his hip. While the activity can be quick with this one, the movement can likewise be sweet and moderate — ideal for apathetic end of the week mornings.

63. **Snow Angel (Bottom's Up):** They get a prime perspective on your derriere. This is testing. Your spouse lies on their back while you ride them confronting endlessly. They lift their legs and fold them over your back to hoist their pelvis so you can enter. They, at that point, snatch your butt to assist you with sliding up and back. They can add a little back rub activity to their hold moreover.

64. **Spin Cycle (Maytag Repair Man):** This is a minor departure from the Hot Seat with your spouse sitting in your lap, yet this time planting yourselves on top of a washing machine set at the most elevated instigator cycle. This substance is imported from {embed-name}. You might have the option to locate a similar substance in another configuration, or you might have the option to discover more data at their site.

65. **Split Missionary:** Here's another missionary variety that permits your mate to dive deep. In split-missionary, you'll keep your legs spread into a split. Split missionary raises the stakes and makes it simple to appreciate the absolute most profound penetration conceivable.

66. **Splitting the Bamboo:** Start by lying on your back and having your spouse jump on top of you to expect the missionary position. At that point, raise one leg and lay it on their shoulder up by their head. Keep the other leg loosened up on the bed. You'll see that with one leg noticeable all around, penetrating

with a penis, finger, or sex toy will feel significantly more profound. In case you're awkward, or your hamstrings are not as adaptable as you'd trusted, request that they stoop all things considered, so they're not giving your raised leg such an extensive amount of stretch.

67. **Spoon (The Sleeper Hold):** Comfortable sex position if your spouse is pregnant or you're substantial. Likewise, ideal for long lovemaking. A great one for nodding off thereafter. You both lie on your sides, confronting a similar bearing, you toward the rear. Your mate twists their knees and pushes their back toward you for simpler penetration to their vagina. Changing the fit of your body will shift the point of passage and help with shaking and pushing.

68. **Spoon, Facing (Sidewinder):** A private up close and personal position that empowers embracing and kissing. This is an ideal position if your spouse is pregnant or both of you had a knee injury since it keeps weight off the body. To get into the position, start by lying on your sides and confronting each other. Your spouse spreads their legs somewhat to permit you to enter them; at that point, shut their legs so the piece of your shaft that is outside can press against their clitoris. It's anything but difficult to kiss from this private vis-à-vis position.

69. **Spooning:** Lots of contacting during sex extends your association, and few positions offer the skin-to-skin contact spoon-style does. This position is overly cuddly and personal, and it likewise makes an altogether different sensation for the two mates. Your shoulders, back, and butt are in close contact with your spouse's middle, and he can stretch around and stroke your bosoms or clitoris for additional sensation.

70. **Spork (Spoon and Fork Combo, Scissoring):** Offers a characteristic scaffold to more imaginative positions. Your spouse lies on their back and raises their correct leg so you can

situate yourself between their legs at a 90-degree point and enter. Their legs will frame the prongs of a spork, a spoon-and-fork utensil. They can do this with you confronting them or confronting their back.

71. **Stairway to Heaven (Step Lively):** This is a minor departure from the Hot Seat with your mate sitting on top of you while you sit on one of the steps of a flight of stairs. Steps offer great seating prospects and a handrail for additional help and lifting influence for them.

72. **Stand and Deliver (The Bicycle):** Stand at the edge of a bed or work area while your spouse lies back and raises their legs to their chest. Their knees are bowed as though they're doing a "bicycling" workout. Get their lower legs and enter them. Push gradually, as the profound entrance might be difficult for them.

73. **Standing O:** While on your knees, let your spouse stand up-right; they should then wrap one of their legs around your shoulder while you eat them out.

74. **Standing Suspended:** In it, as you may figure, the man is standing, and the lady is suspended, her legs folded over his thighs and his hands measuring her butt. This is the most troublesome situation for a couple to keep up for any time. For individuals who need to give this position a test drive, they can think about utilizing it as a momentary move starting with one area then onto the next.

75. **Standing Tiger, Crouching Dragon:** Doing it from behind gets a ton more blazing with this basic variety. Bow on the bed (or sofa, or feasting table, or floor, or any raised surface), and let your standing spouse enter you from behind. This permits them to hit unexpected points in comparison to if you were simply twisted around. The sensation will change depending on how far

separated you place your legs. Play with opening your legs more extensive and smaller to discover what feels best to you.

76. **Standing Wheelbarrow:** This one will truly get the blood hurrying to your head and is a simple accomplishment for committed yogis. Accept descending doggy position, and afterward, let your mate tenderly get your legs and fold them over their abdomen. You'll uphold yourself with your arms, and for added uphold, they'll additionally hold you up by your hips.

77. **Standing:** With the two spouses standing and confronting one another or away from one another (with a divider for help), the individual with the vulva spreads their legs, while the individual with the penis or dildo infiltrates them. Contingent upon the stature distinction, this will include both the vulva proprietor directing the penis proprietor inside them, just as some changing and straightening out of the standing positions.

78. **Swiss Ball Blitz (Romper Room):** Have a ball in your exercise room? Utilize a security ball to add some bob to The Hot Seat. Sit ready with your feet on the floor. Let your spouse back up onto you, sitting between your legs. Roll and bob to it.

79. **Table Top:** You don't need to do this one on a table — any surface that hits your mate at groin stature will do. Have them enter you while you're sitting or lying at the edge of a table, counter, or possibly your bed. This position is incredible for up close and personal activity. Besides, if both of you are radically various statures, this is an incredible alternative since it puts you both at similar tallness.

80. **Tap Dance:** Lie on one side with one leg expanded and the other bowed. With one hand, tenderly isolate and hold your labia to the sides, and apply a little drop of lube to your uncovered clitoris. At that point, with the contrary hand, start tapping tenderly on it. Tapping, rather than scouring, can create snappy

and serious uproars for the individuals who find direct incitement excessively extraordinary.

81. **The 69:** No entrance is vital for this vibe great sex position — simply shared oral sex. Either spouse can be on top or on base. Line yourselves up head to toe and delight each other all the while.

82. **The Amazon:** In this position, the lady squats over her spouse, situated on the rear of his legs. His legs are moved up toward her chest, and she is squatting with her feet level. This position should likewise be possible with the lady turned around or potentially stooping.

83. **The Arch:** The explanation behind the Arch is that it requires the infiltrating spouse to accomplish the aerobatic work. All the collector needs to do is ride and squat — something that requires some thigh quality yet little adaptability.

84. **The Babysitter:** This sitter is basically face-sitting light. The individual getting oral sex rides the supplier and brings down themselves onto the provider's mouth (as would occur in a face-sitting position); however, the recipient at that point inclines forward and underpins themselves with their hands. This gives the supplier all the more space to breathe while as yet bearing the cost of the free access from beneath.

85. **The Ballet Dancer (Get a Leg Up):** You stand confronting each other. Your spouse raises one of their legs and folds it over your hindquarters or thigh and maneuvers you into them with their leg.

86. **The Bouncy Chair:** First, advise your mate to get down on their knees (this is fun as of now!). Have their bow with their butt behind them and the chunks of their feet on the ground. Ride their lap, confronting them with your feet level on the floor on one or the other side of their legs. When you're in position

(and their penis or tie-on is inside you), skip on the wads of your feet to control the mood and entrance. The nearness will make for some scrumptious cozy time.

87. **The Caboose:** While they sit on the bed or a seat, back yourself into their lap and spoon one another while situated. You can't see your spouse during this sex position, which means fantasizing is simpler and can add to the energy. Fix the muscles of your pelvic floor so you can grasp them and keep them hard AF or stimulate their clitoris.

88. **The Cat (Coital Alignment Technique):** The CAT is fundamentally the same as the missionary position aside from your body is situated farther up and aside. Rather than being chest to chest, your chest is close to your spouse's shoulders. Have them twist their legs around 45 degrees to tilt their hips up. This makes the base of your shaft keep in touch with the clitoris.

89. **The Chairman:** Your mate sits on the edge of the bed, and you sit on them, confronting endlessly. This sex position will hit the spot, as in, your G-spot. In the chairman, you can utilize your hands to animate their scrotum, perineum, or clitoris. Carry your knees closer to your chest, supporting your feet on the bed.

90. **The Chairwoman:** Find a seat (ideally one without arms) and cause your spouse to sit their stripped self down. At that point, sit down on their lap, confronting endlessly from them, and lead their hand to any place it is you like to be contacted. At the point when you can't take the prodding any longer, reposition yourself so that they're within you while you're actually sitting on them. Urge them to continue contacting you while you move to and fro until either of you peak.

91. **The Champagne Room:** This is so near the Chairwoman, yet there's one unobtrusive (however particular) contrast. Instead of riding your spouse, keep your legs shut and your knees together.

This welcomes on an altogether extraordinary inclination and keeps things super close.

92. **The Cradle:** Let your spouse sit as though they're doing the butterfly stretch. At that point, confronting ceaselessly from them, move into their lap, and have them lift you up — knees twisted, as though you're doing youngster's posture to the air. Since you're completely without hands (appendages free, truly), your spouse can assume absolute responsibility for the profundity and speed of entrance — leaving you totally accommodating.

93. **The Cross:** First, the individual with the penis or dildo lies nonchalantly on their side. You know, as though they were modeling for a photograph. They can either prop their head up with their arm or lay it on their all-encompassing arm. Next, the individual with the vulva kind of shimmies themselves into place as though they're perched on their mate's lap. At that point, they (the individual with the vulva) wraps their legs over their spouse's hips so they can be entered.

94. **The Double Dip:** For this one, you'll have to bring in reinforcement. You will require one individual with a dildo or penis and two individuals with vulvas. To start with, the two individuals with the vulvas need to get into fundamental missionary, while the individual with the penis or dildo jumps on their knees and enters the two individuals with vulvas — independently obviously — except if there's a twofold dildo circumstance included.

95. **The Elevator (The Bees Knees):** Great for out-of-room fellatio. Your spouse bows before you, covering their teeth with their lips and surrounding your glans with their mouth. They then gradually cylinder their lips here and there on your shaft, exchanging speeds and infrequently halting to move their tongue over and around your head.

96. **The Fusion (Getting a Leg Up):** Quicker climaxes for your spouse; simpler movements. From the Spider, your spouse can lift their legs onto your shoulders, which expands the solid pressure that progresses the climax succession. By raising their butt off the bed, it'll be simpler for them to push and granulate around and around.

97. **The Good Ex:** Sit on the bed, confronting each other with legs forward. Lift your mate's right leg over your left and lift your right leg over their left. Meet up so they can enter you. Presently both of you lie back, your legs shaping an X. Slow, relaxed gyrations supplant pushing. Delayed moderate sex that will fabricate your excitement. Shallow pushes invigorate the sensitive spots in the top of their penis on the off chance that they have one.

98. **The Greasy Spoon:** Assume the spoon position, yet lift one leg! You can prop it up with pads or take on the situation on the lounge chair (where you would then be able to snare your foot over the back rest).

99. **The G-Whiz (The Shoulder Holder, The Anvil):** Your spouse lies on their back. You stoop between their legs and raise them, resting their calves over your shoulders. Rock them in a side-to-side and here-and-there movement to bring the head and shaft of your penis in direct contact with the front mass of their vagina. Since this point considers profound infiltration, pushed gradually from the outset, try not to cause distress.

100. **The Hashtag (The Intersection):** It is a pound sign, all things considered (get it?). To take on the position; lie on your side while your spouse bows confronting you and lift up your top leg (like the scissors position). In this position, the lady lays on her side. The man, likewise on his side, is behind her with both of his legs between her legs. Together, they structure an X shape, subsequently the name.

101. **The Helicopter:** As the getting spouse gets outfit on all fours, the entering mate floats on, infiltrating them from a cross-breed board/handstand position. It's muddled whether the spouses remain static and just push from this position or whether they turn their bodies to copy the development of a helicopter. In any case, the position is equivalent amounts of bonkers and charming — and it's certain to make them start to perspire.

102. **The Hill:** In the Hill, the accepting spouse basically remains against the divider, while the infiltrating mate turns over and enters them from a handstand position. At that point, the collector ought to likely advance in with force and deal with the pushing circumstance (yet not very forcefully, in case they overturn their hand-standing spouse). On the off chance that the top can all the while handstand and push, they merit overwhelming applause.

103. **The Hot Seat (The Sofa, The Man Chair):** Sit on the edge of the bed or on a seat with your feet on the floor. Your mate dismisses and backs up onto you, sitting between your legs. They can ride to and fro by pushing off the seat arms or squeezing up with their feet. They can control the point of the section by curving their back and squeezing their bum into your crotch. While doggy style is about your predominance, The Hot Seat places your spouse steering the ship. Furthermore, that makes it extraordinary compared to other sex positions for both of you.

104. **The iPhone X:** This move praises that greater is better. Lie on your back and push your hips up into an extension (keep your head and neck on the bed while supporting yourself with your shoulders). Your spouse remains on the bed, riding you, holding your hips up. It's a move up to your standard daily practice without a doubt, yet kindly don't call technical support if things go astray.

105. **The Laptop:** There's nothing closer than eye-to-eye, slow, profound infiltration sex. This one includes a touch of adaptability. The mate entering with their penis or toy sits in a (durable!) seat with their feet level on the floor, while the other spouse sits on their lap, confronting them. Rest the backs of your knees on your spouse's shoulders and your calves and feet on or over the rear of a seat.

106. **The Lazy Man:** Place cushions despite your mate's good faith and have them sit on the bed with legs outstretched. Presently ride their midsection, feet on the bed. Curve your knees to bring down yourself onto them, utilizing one hand to coordinate the penis or tie on in. Just by pushing on the wads of your feet and delivering, you can raise and lower yourself onto the shaft as gradually or as fast however you see fit.

107. **The Lean-In:** Sometimes, keeping it straightforward is the ideal approach. Lie on your back and permit your spouse to go down on you while likewise infiltrating you with a finger or sex toy simultaneously. Such an overachiever.

108. **The Little Dipper:** For the Little Dipper, the individual on top uses either a bed, sofa, or seat to lift themselves over their spouse. The individual on base at that point embeds his penis into the top's vagina or butt. The top, at that point, does rear arm muscles plunges to go here and there on their mate's penis. Whenever done accurately, you should be in a T-shape arrangement.

109. **The Lotus:** Have the mate with the penis or dildo sit with their legs crossed — you know, as you did when you were a child and it was storytime. Next, the individual with the vulva brings down themselves into their spouse's lap and onto them while folding their legs and arms over their spouse's body. At that point, you start to shake together.

110. **The Mermaid:** Lie down with your butt agreed with the edge of the bed or table (place a pad under your hips if you need more stature). At that point, set your legs on the right track out of sight, calve together like a mermaid's tail. The embedding spouse can enter with a penis, finger, or sex toy.

111. **The Octopus:** You lie on your back and position yourself in the middle of your spouse's open legs (they'll be sitting up). Scooch yourself closer to them, place every one of your legs over their shoulders and have them embed themselves into you. From that point, remove it with delicate pushes. Keep it without rushing, however, since it's simple for the penis or tie-on to sneak out in this position.

112. **The Om:** Let your mate sit leg over the leg and move on board. Fold your legs over their midsection, and rock to and fro for tantric-style sex. This up close and personal position is unimaginably cozy since you can stare at your sweetheart.

113. **The Om:** Your spouse sits leg over leg (yoga/pretzel-style), you sit in their lap, confronting them. Fold your legs over them and embrace each other for help. Best for tantric sex. Shaking, not pushing, is the key with regards to this personal position.

114. **The Pinball Wizard:** Lie on your back and lift your hips up as though you were in an extension position (leaving your shoulders on the bed). Your mate can hold your hips up as they enter you from a bowing position. It permits your mate simpler admittance to animate your clitoris and back rub the mons pubis. Hurl one leg against their shoulder for a more profound penetration.

115. **The Pretzel (The Pretzel Dip, The Camel Ride):** Kneel and ride their left leg while they're lying on their left side. Your spouse will twist their correct leg around the correct side of your midriff, which will give you admittance to enter their vagina. For some individuals with vulvas, back passage harms their backs.

This sex position permits them to serenely relax while appreciating profound penetration.

116. **The Seashell:** Lie back with your legs raised as far as possible up and your lower legs crossed behind your own head. They enter you from a missionary position. Your hands are allowed to work your clitoris as you should. Have them "enjoy some real success," scouring their pubic bone against your clitoris, or "ride low," straightforwardly invigorating your G-spot with the top of the penis, the tie on, a dildo, or a finger.

117. **The Sideways Straddle:** Who needs their clitoris stimulated? You do! Probably the best situation for clitoral incitement is the sideways ride, and it's anything but difficult to do. Let your mate, together with the penis or dildo, set down level on their back, with one leg loosened up and one leg bowed at the knee. At that point, confronting endlessly from your spouse, slide yourself down onto them, so you enter from the back while having the option to utilize their leg to invigorate your clit.

118. **The Snake:** Lie down on your stomach, and let your spouse rests on top of you and slide in from behind. This position considers super-profound penetration and a cozy fit that can feel extraordinary for you and your mate.

119. **The Socket:** From switch cowgirl, have them twist right forward, broadening their legs right back. They should be supporting their body by laying on their elbows as though they were holding a board.

120. **The Spider:** You both can even now keep in touch while seeing the activity in the middle of everyone's attention. Both of you are situated on the bed with legs toward each other, arms back to help yourselves. Presently move together, and they move onto you. Their hips will be between your spread legs, their knees

twisted and feet outside of your hips and level on the bed. Presently rock to and fro.

121. **Standing 69:** One individual stands upstanding, and the other goes into a handstand while the former holds them. This ought to permit you both to arrive at one another's mischievous pieces, however, you may need to stop it before all the blood hurries to your head. This may be even more a "fair to state we did it" sort of position, truly.

122. **The Standing Dragon (Crouching Tiger, Hidden Serpent):** Stand and enter your spouse from behind as they present down on the ground on the edge of the bed and curve their back to lift their posterior.

123. **The Standing Slide:** In the Standing Slide, the entering spouse ought to hurry in a bad position until just their head and shoulders are touching the ground (the remainder of their body should be as straight as could reasonably be expected, inclining toward the divider). The other mate should move toward them, confronting their body and getting as close as could be expected under the circumstances. The accepting spouse should then spread their legs apart and squat until they arrive at their spouse's penis or lash on. From that point, they can control the profundity and speed of infiltration.

124. **The Superman:** Pretend you're doing doggy style, with your legs folded over your spouse's body. Besides, rather than them bowing and you lying forward, they're standing, reclining, and you're suspended in mid-air.

125. **The Swing:** For it, the man leans back on his back with his feet on the ground and knees up, at that point raises his hips off the floor in a lower-body connection. The lady is situated on top of him.

126. **The Twerk:** The twerk adds on to turn around cowgirl. Accept the converse cowgirl position and lean forward, laying your arms on their thighs. At that point, just utilize the twerking movement (curve your back and rock to and fro, popping your goods all over) to engage in sexual relations.

127. **The Worm:** This is another variety of Missionary; however, it has the lady on top and confronting the man's feet. The two mates have their legs spread in an X shape. Start this situation with the lady situated on top, at that point step by step inclining forward.

128. **The X Position (Crisscross):** Prolonged moderate sex to assemble excitement. Shallow pushes animate the sensitive spots in the top of your penis. Sit on the bed, confronting each other with legs forward. Lift your correct leg over their left, and they lift their correct leg over your left. Meet up so you can enter. Presently both of you lie back, with your legs shaping an X. Slow, relaxed gyrations supplant pushing.

129. **The Zombie:** The Zombie is the ideal situation for those of us who are adaptable, however not very adaptable. (Would you be able to twist around and contact your toes easily with your knees bowed? You can deal with this.) In this collapsed type of 69, one spouse sits on the ground while different stands over them and twists down. This puts the standing spouse's genitalia upfront for the sitting spouse and the sitting mate's genitalia upfront for the standing spouse. Everybody wins.

130. **Tigress:** Think to turn around cowgirl with a wind. Let your spouse rests; at that point, you sit on top of them, confronting endlessly. Presently reach back and place one hand on their chest. Use your hand to settle yourself as you go all over. This permits you to have unlimited authority over the speed and profundity of infiltration. You can likewise have them put their hands on your midsection if you discover you need a lift.

131. **Upstanding Citizen:** You ride them, folding your legs over their body (they keep their knees opened and thighs spread somewhat). They stand and supporting you in their arms. You can begin in the bed and have them get you without separating. Or, on the other hand, for the really striking, you can jump on board from a standing position!

132. **Valedictorian:** Get in the missionary position. Then, raise your legs and expand them straight till you get a "V" shape. This takes into consideration great body contact with the clit. Take a stab at holding onto your lower legs. It can allow you steadiness and an additional stretch to help the sensation.

133. **Waterfall (Head Rush):** Move to the edge of the bed and lie back with your head and shoulders on the floor as your mate rides you. The blood will race to your head, making stunning sensations upon climax.

134. **Weak in the Knees:** Similar to situated oral, you and your spouse need to choose who's getting and giving first. For hell's sake, you can even flip a coin and settle on the choice much simpler. At that point, one spouse rides the other mate's face so they can get oral.

135. **Wheelbarrow:** Get on all fours and have them get you by the pelvis. At that point, hold their midsection with your thighs. Besides being an astounding arm exercise, this male-prevailing sex position considers further entrance. Have a go at laying on a table or the side of the bed and offer your arms a reprieve.

136. **Widely Opened:** Lie level on your back. Let your spouse stoop on the edge of the bed with their knees somewhat separated, and fold your legs over their midriff. At that point, raise your hips and pelvis by curving your back giving, your spouse a magnificent view. Have them uphold you by holding the little of your back while they do the pushing.

137. **X Marks the Spot:** While the individual with the vulva lays on their back — a table is entirely wonderful for this one — they lift their advantages and cross them at the lower legs or knees, whatever feels best. With their advantages, they cooperate with the penis or dildo while in a standing position, penetrate them, while using the legs of the vulva proprietor as an influence to pull themselves in more profound. It's an extraordinary situation for individuals with more modest penises.

138. **Yab yum (sitting with legs crossed):** Yab yum is a Tantric sex position and it involves sitting down and facing each other. The man should sit upstanding with the legs either extended before his body or crossed. The female partner sits on his lap while facing his direction and with legs wrapped around his hips. Their hands can be folded around each other as well. Then, each of them can start nestling, kissing, and touching every area of their partner's body.

139. **Yourself on the Shelf (The Bicycle):** The woman can sit directly on the edge of a seat or bed. The man stands in front, facing her, and then enters. At that point, the woman would fold her legs around the man. Then, the man stands up-right, wrapping his hands around her back to help his mate.

Doggy Style

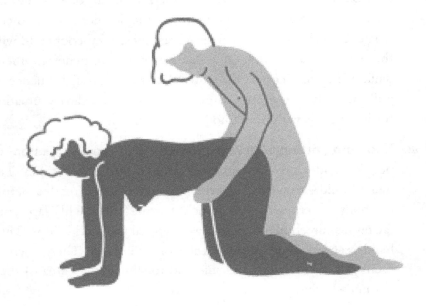

Albeit most couples have likely attempted to zest things up by changing to doggy style occasionally, you presumably aren't exploring different avenues regarding it enough. Studies have demonstrated that practically 30% of ladies incline toward doggy style over the other customary sex positions, and different reviews show that doggy style may be the most mainstream style among the two sexual orientations. Indeed, it very well may be the best situation for hitting the G-spot.

Doggy style gets a terrible rep in light of the fact that there's no eye-to-eye contact and it's not seen as being as 'cozy' as, state, the missionary position. The thing is, confronting endlessly from one another isn't really a terrible thing. In the event that you actually feel hesitant about the face you make during sex, doggy style can cause you to feel allowed to let free.

Besides, if you preclude doggy-style sex, you can truly pass up a portion of the incredible possible advantages of the position (like G-spot and A-spot incitement, bosom play, and the sky is the limit from there). That is the reason, if you have a prepared and willing spouse, you can make a few changes to the doggy-style sex position and offer it one more opportunity.

Doggy style is the point at which one spouse is situated behind the other and penetrates their vagina or butt from behind, using a toy, penis, or finger. Commonly, this occurs with the getting mate situated in a hands-and-knees position down on the ground. Yet, you've really got alternatives.

Doggy style is a staggeringly adjustable back section position. Doggy should be possible standing, bowing, lying on your side or your stomach, while twisted around the sofa, in a bad position; whatever makes you excited.

On the off chance that you've checked doggy style out yet haven't felt like you're arriving at your most extreme delight, it may very well involve fitting a couple of subtleties to suit you and your spouse's requirements.

- It's ideal for stimulating the G-spot.

Named after the primary specialist to depict it in clinical writing, Ernst Gräfenber, the G-spot is a penny-sized joy point that is around two inches deep on the front vaginal divider. You've presumably heard you can discover this spot by making a come-here stroking movement with your fingers inside your vagina — this is valid. However, it can likewise be animated through doggy-style sex.

Your spouse will have the option to best hit your G-Spot if you bring down your middle toward the bed. Along these lines, let your chest area unwind and request to let your mate be pushed moderate and shallow. Keep in mind, the G-spot is just an inch, or a few, inside the vaginal divider, so no compelling reason to go penetrating for treasure.

- A-spot stimulation is not left out.

A couple of inches further than the previously mentioned G-detect, the front fornix erogenous zone (as it used to be called) is found somewhere inside the vagina between the cervix and the bladder. The point of section during doggy-style sex empowers the profound penetration which is important for invigorating this delight point.

Contingent upon the length of your spouse's penis/dildo/finger, they might have the option to stimulate your A-spot while you're down on the ground. If not, dropping onto your elbows will open you up considerably more and permit your spouse to dive further into your body. Another choice: Lay level on your stomach and let your mate lie on top of you, similar to two stacked flapjacks.

A few people may encounter an "A-spot climax" from profound penetration, while others may have a mixed climax if they consolidate this sensation with some clitoral consideration.

- You can control how deep it gets.

On the off chance that you feel apprehensive about giving the doggy style a go explicitly because you discover profound entrance awkward or even difficult, uplifting news: There are approaches to appreciate the situation without all the profundities. Anal sex ought to never, under any circumstance, be agonizing. If it is, you're not going moderate enough or utilizing enough lube.

- Your butt is not left out of the activity.

It's an extraordinary situation for anal sex. To attempt it, lube up your butt and your spouse's condom-clad penis/dildo. At that point, have them press the tip against your butthole and gradually apply pressure while you press once more into the sensation. Numerous people with vulvas are amazed by how great this can feel on the off chance that they start smooth and moderate. For what reason does it feel so great? Anal penetration can, by implication, animate the A-spot.

- You're in an extraordinary situation for oral sex.

You can get into the doggy-style beneficiary position and renounce the entrance. (Indeed truly!) Being down on the ground takes incredible access for your spouse to perform cunnilingus or give you an edge work.

Notwithstanding by and large amazing feeling, this kind of oral play before sex can help make the doggy style position or any sex position, so far as that is concerned, more pleasant. The vagina normally grows as you get stirred, so foreplay is basic for joy.

- It doesn't need a bed.

On the off chance that you and your mate love quick ones or engaging in sexual relations in unpredictable areas (read: *not* in the room), doggy style — explicitly standing doggy style — is awesome. You can do it in the shower, over the restroom sink, in a flight of stairs, a separated lift, an upkeep/coat wardrobe, or... well, anyplace.

- It can be really close.

You probably won't know it from watching the doggy style in pornography, yet it can be more associated than animalistic. Let your spouse encompassed you from behind, practically like you're spooning so their arms are wrapped immovably around you. Make it more private still by laying level on the bed so that every last trace of your back is covered by your skin.

You could consider setting a mirror before you for an all the more genuine and crude bend on doggy style. Locking eyes through your appearance can elevate closeness, and watching yourselves play can help excitement. It's practically similar to featuring in and viewing a sensual film simultaneously. Furthermore, if your spouse shuts their eyes in a snapshot of rapture, you will observe exactly the amount they appreciate it and you.

69

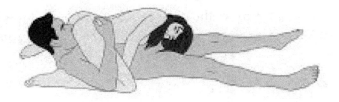

There are not many sexual positions more polarizing than 69. A considerable lot of us attempted the exemplary position a couple of times in secondary school and early school yet immediately surrendered it, deciding that it's a great deal of off-kilter work for the negligible prize. Additionally, the individual better at giving oral giving winds up rebuffed for their boss abilities since the recipient begins groaning boisterously, taking a break from orally satisfying their mate. That is not how 69 functions! To do the 69 sex position effectively, the two individuals included need to give and get oral all the while.

In case you're somebody who needs to simply zero in on accepting delight, that is thoroughly fine. You can appreciate being the collector without zeroing in on giving — yet then 69 isn't appropriate for you. The equivalent is valid on the off chance that you simply need to give oral. It tends to be trying to accomplish your best work on another person on the off chance that they're additionally pleasuring you. You may likewise be somebody who essentially doesn't care for getting oral yet cherishes giving it. Once more, this is thoroughly fine — whatever puts a smile on your face — yet then you should pass on 69-ing and settle on another wonderful sex position, all things considered.

Presently, concerning the individuals who like 69; they frequently truly like it. They like that the two spouses can get and appreciate joy simultaneously. The vast majority, who like 69, have placed in the work to become geniuses at the convoluted position. They don't hurry into it. They discover a style that works for the two of them, where doesn't stress their necks to get where they have to go.

So, we should discuss 69 and its numerous versions.

- Classic 69

Two individuals adjust themselves so that every individual's mouth is close to the next's private parts. This is finished by having one individual rests on their back. One lies on top of them with their knees riding their spouse's head. The two individuals would then be able to perform oral sex on each other. In other gender spouses, the lady is normally the individual on top, while the man is on his back. Use a cushion or a sex wedge in case you're battling to reach or wind up stressing your neck or another piece of your body.

- Inverted 69

It's equivalent to the classic variation; in any case, rather than the lady is on top, the man is. While not natural in the variety itself, the altered 69 position will, in general, be a more unpleasant encounter. It's an ideal situation for ladies who like to deepthroat because with the man on top, he has more control of his pushing capacity and can go significantly harder and more profound down the throat.

- Sideways 69

Instead of situating one on top of the other, the two members are lying on their sides. If you're battling to arrive at one another's private parts with the exemplary 69, sideways 69 might be the position for you. I would say it makes it simpler to arrive at everything. It additionally requires less work for the individual who's generally on top. While on top, you're regularly on your knees and, in any event, one elbow, which can be difficult for extensive periods.

- Squatting 69

Instead of having your mate lie on top of you, have them squat over you. This will require lower back, glute, and quad quality, and adaptability, yet on the off chance that they have it, it's a pleasant minor departure from the work of art. The squat variety additionally takes into account better ass slapping.

- The Standing 69

Rather than lying on a level surface, you really hold your spouse up-side-down while you're standing. You will feel like a divine being in case you're ready to pull this off. Unless you are a muscle daddy, chances are you won't have the solidarity to get your spouse securely. That is the reason this position is ideal when your mate is especially dainty.

- Penetrative 69

Notwithstanding orally animating your spouse, utilize either your fingers or a sex toy to enter them. On the off chance that your spouse has a vagina, you can lick/suck their clitoris while carefully entering her vagina. Or then again, if your mate is into it, you can eat their vagina while you finger their rear-end (or bad habit a-versa). You can do this with men, as well. While being blown, let your spouse rub your prostate for more exceptional delight. With interior incitement, delight rises dramatically for the two players included.

- Analingus 69

While we're on the subject of anal comprehensive 69 variations, you can simply eat out your spouse's goods only. Or then again, a variety that is basic among two men is the point at which the "base" (the one getting anal) blows their mate, where the top (the one who will embed his penis into his spouse) eats out their spouse's rear-end. It's a type of foreplay to release and heat up the base for penetrative anal sex. If you're into anal and additionally prostate play, this is for you.

- Threesome 69 (otherwise known as The Triangle)

Well, most importantly, you have to acquire an exceptional third for the trio 69. While lying on your side with your spouses in a triangle arrangement, each mate performs oral on the following individual. In this position, you will perform oral on one spouse and get oral from the other. It's hot to have a third individual in on all the good times. It's additionally a trio position that is similarly comprehensive of all gatherings included.

Reverse Cowgirl

On the off chance that you realize how to do an ordinary cowgirl position (face your spouse and ride them with a knee on one or the other side of their hips); at that point, you realize how to do the reverse cowgirl. You should simply flip it and converse it.

Everything about reverse cowgirl seems like it was worked to stir your wild side. However, in principle, it can get somewhat abnormal. All things considered, it tends to be dubious to sort out some way to move a smooth ride; at that point, there's likewise the entire goods in-your-mate's-face part of the position.

However, the invert cowgirl position additionally permits you to take the rules, which means you're in charge. Be that as it may, how does the reverse cowgirl position work?

Step-by-step instructions to Sit on top of your mate, confronting their feet; at that point, have your spouse twist his legs or keep them straight. In any case, hang on close and begin going here and there to discover what feels better.

What's so extraordinary about it?

- Visual incitement

The second you change to this situation after the customary cowgirl, your man gets totally invigorated if he, as of now, isn't. Men appreciate seeing you from behind (no big surprise, doggy style is one of the most loved situations for some men), and this position offers you simply that.

- Lady in force

If you like taking control or your man loves to be agreeable, at that point, this is the best position. You have full oversight on the point, the movement, the profundity, everything. You have the reins in your grasp and you can make your man insane because no other position makes a lady hotter than this one.

- Hands-free

Since both of you have your hands free, there's so much you can do with them. You can play with his balls or give him a decent thigh rub while he can beat you or take a stab at stimulating your clit or play with your boobs. The delight is raised in this position.

- Better view

Do it before the mirror, and you'll have a stunning perspective on your body while your man is blessed to receive your excellent bends and behind. This is likewise a superb situation for ladies with little boobs who feel odd in cowgirl or different positions.

- More profound infiltration

The opposite cowgirl encourages you to hit the G-spot just consummately. The entrance is profound, and the point gives you a superior vaginal sensation as well. This position permits men to last somewhat more in bed since they are totally loose and consequently is a finished mutual benefit for ladies.

- Gives you a simple change from schedule

The position isn't excessively convoluted like a portion of the difficult Kamasutra positions, and you don't should be very adaptable or bend yourself into some awkward posture! In this way, you can attempt it with the least exertion and hotshot your abilities in bed and let the man unwind and appreciate for some time.

The key is getting settled regardless of whether it implies getting settled with being somewhat awkward.

A great deal of the tests for ladies during sex is how they see their own bodies and they stress. However, with reverse cowgirl — or any sex position besides, there's an open door for ladies to comprehend that what turns men on isn't the alleged flawlessness of the body, yet a lady who truly is okay with herself.

You can quit agonizing over what you look like and get completely centered around the sensations and causing the sex to feel stunning. Without stressing over your exhibition, you'll ideally not hesitate to let your hips move as you undulate and push in all the manners that vibe best to you.

Furthermore, with you accountable for the position, it permits you to shake things up with dynamic force in your love affair. Playing with these various parts of manly and ladylike energy can be an approach to assist us with getting unstuck from our standard functions in bed.

Spooning

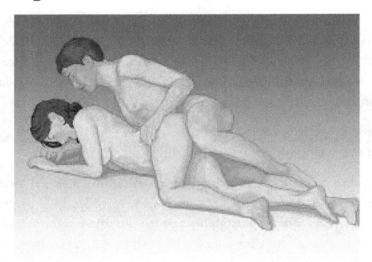

Spooning alludes to lying on your side with a spouse lying on their side and twisting up behind you, emulating spoons that consistently fit together. Individuals have been spooning for quite a long time, as apparent from memorable fine art portraying sexual grasps and positions between same-sex and heterosexual couples.

What are the advantages of spooning?

There are some intuitive components affecting everything with regards to why spooning will, in general, trigger such compelling feelings. The biggest organ we have on our bodies is our skin, and the base inclination to have skin-to-skin contact for most people is because of our craving to be relieved, ameliorated, and cherished. Individuals appreciate spooning because it's a method to be near your mate in an erotic way that is not really sexual. There aren't an excessive number of different approaches to truly interface with your spouse that doesn't include sex or kissing.

Post-sex spooning is an approach to proceed with the exceptional closeness experienced during the climax. There are numerous ways we have intercourse with one another, with the demonstration of sex being only one of them. Spooning and holding each other is a type of communicating love and a profound feeling of thinking about one another.

- Spooning improves unwinding and hormone discharge.

At the point when you spoon with a mate, you'll notice your breath start to slow, develop, and sync. In addition to the fact that this feels unwinding, yet it likewise triggers an arrival of oxytocin, a hormone, and synapse which scientists accept is connected to passion of holding and sexual excitement.

Participating in spooning can likewise deliver dopamine which is liable for remuneration and inspiration in the cerebrum, and serotonin which settles temperament. These synthetic substances delivered during spooning can likewise diminish pressure, improve rest, and straightforwardness torment by delivering endorphins, the body's common painkillers.

This all adds to helping our sensory system unwind. We are designed to interact as individuals, and the actual touch and embracing that happens during spooning brings down our pulse and makes an impression on our bodies that it's okay to unwind and give up.

- Spooning assists couples with feeling intimate.

A few specialists have even discovered that utilizing spooning procedures in their meetings can assist couples with feeling intimate. At the point when I'm working with couples, I'll have them attempt this in the workplace by setting a clock for five minutes and requesting that they rest together, with however much of their bodies contacting as could reasonably be expected, with no plan other than to see what's going on in their bodies. Before 5 minutes' over, most couples report feeling nearer sincerely and keen on raising their actual association.

- It's a substitute type of closeness.

Spooning is a decent option for individuals who experience issues with eye-to-eye connection after sex. The position offers another option, where within spoon, the spouse is so near the other they can hear their breathing, feel the other's pulse, and be held by — with no interest on that enormous spoon mate.

- It's a simple segue to intercourse.

In any case, spooning can likewise be a sex position, one that can be effortlessly fused in case you're feeling somewhat drained or lethargic. During sex, the little spoon is the getting spouse, and the huge spoon is the one entering, either with their penis or a lash on.

The little spoon can manage their spouse while curving to get the correct point. Contingent upon every individual's size, there might be some changing required going up, down, or forward to get an agreeable fit. The two mates can add to the pushing, and the two spouses can add to invigorating the little spoon, so they are getting stimulated remotely and inside utilizing hands, fingers, or potentially toys.

Sitting

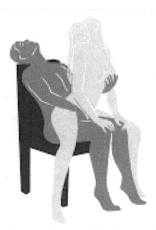

Huge numbers of us consider sex objections in pretty twofold terms: We're either doing it some place truly ribald, or we're getting it on in a room. There's a great deal of room between those two limits; however, we don't generally endeavor into it. Furthermore, that is a disgrace, since that center ground is basically asking to be investigated.

The beds are incredible. They're extraordinary to rest, relax, stare at the TV, eat in and shake the pieces out of, and an exemplary scene for getting it on. However, bed sex, while extraordinary, can likewise get a little old if it's the main sex scene you're frequenting. That is the reason it's useful to wander out and take your sexing to another area.

While for some gutsy people that implies nature or an extravagant lodging in another city, all you truly require to shake things up are some sex moves to attempt in a seat — and a consistent seat to destroy them. The open door for sexploration and zestiness is only a room away.

Truth is stranger than fiction; seat sex positions proliferate—and they don't request that much from you. You don't need to do anything confounded or hazardous getting trapped in the demonstration. You're essentially welcome to deliver your sex schedule somewhat more energizing by moving to a marginally extraordinary corner of your home.

The seat sex position is probably as tremendous and changed as some others. Since there are a ton of approaches to do it on a seat. You can have comfortable, cozy seat sex. You can try aerobatic seat sex. You can have relaxed, apathetic seat sex. You can be vivacious, adoring, forceful, laidback — and each shade of dim in the middle. Seat sex runs a similar extent of feelings and encounters as some other sort of sex. Since, well, it's simply sex — that turns out to be occurring on a seat. What's pleasant? Although seat sex isn't uncommon or selective, it actually feels fun, energizing, and extraordinary. It's as yet a break from the standard. Seat sex is a decent update that we don't have to travel significant distances or go through extravagant measures of money to experience. We can just investigate space in our home in a shiny new manner. It may not be an all-out excursion, yet it's, in any event, a smidgen of a departure — and one that is certain to be a wide range of fun.

If you think seat sex is restricting, reconsider because these positions run the extent from simple, loose, and ideal for moderate lovemaking. Right to so extreme and heart-beating that you have your cardio covered for the week. Whatever your speed (in a real sense and allegorically), these seat sex positions have you covered. All things considered, here are some situated hot time positions to add to your collection. Cautioning: Some of these are so hot, you may fail to remember you even have a bed.

1. Roosted Pleasure Position

Of all the seat positions, this one is likely the simplest to accomplish, so attempt to truly move slowly and appreciate. To get into this position, the penetrating spouse sits in the seat, and the getting spouse sits on their lap, being entered from behind. This position likewise has the advantage of leaving both mate's hands allowed to investigate.

2. Living on the edge

For a further developed seat position, check this one out, however, know that it takes a reasonable piece of equilibrium and solidarity to accomplish. To accept this position, the infiltrating partner sits back in the seat with legs immovably planted on the ground. The getting spouse at that point starts by riding their spouse and afterward cautiously reclining. With the help of the infiltrating mate, the accepting spouse's legs are then positioned on their spouse's shoulders. This is extraordinary for moderate, delicate, tantric style sex, although it requires a ton of center quality.

3. The Giddy-Up Position

This position doesn't need much adaptability or chest area quality; however, it will get your heart hustling. To accomplish this position, start with entering mate sitting close to the edge of the seat with legs outstretched. The getting spouse would then be able to ride them. The two spouses would then be able to recline marginally, and the accepting spouse can utilize the shaking of their legs to control the speed and profundity of infiltration.

4. Bow And-Deliver Position

For another position that is somewhat more unwinding yet very hot, attempt the Kneel-And-Deliver. To get into this position, the accepting mate plunks down on the edge of the seat, and the infiltrating spouse stoops before them inclines marginally back and lays on their hamstrings. The accepting spouse, at that point, folds their legs over their mate's hips so they can be in charge of the pushing.

5. Got-Your-(Chair) Back Position

Not all seat positions must be situated. Truth be told, one of the most sweltering and least demanding of all is standing. Essentially, the accepting spouse twists forward, using the seat as help while the infiltrating spouse enters behind. Investigate which points feel best by utilizing both the back and the seat of the seat to help you at various statures. Trust me, when you hit your own sweet spot, you'll know it.

Out of nowhere, having the partner haul your seat out for you has taken on a totally different (and hot) means. Try not to be reluctant to fan out of your room and check one of these situated situations out. (In any case, perhaps work up to the Living-On-The-Edge position, simply saying.)

Standing (Suspended and Face to Face)

At the point when most couples have intercourse, they regularly do it on a level plane on a bed. Hello, we have no issue with that. It's difficult to beat the solace of solid bedding and a few fleecy pads. Also, when the activity is finished, you can essentially float off to rest.

In any case, there's a solid case to be made for escaping the sack — and getting up on your feet. Sex standing up may not generally be actually simple. Yet, carrying it out this way carries curiosity to your sexual coexistence, and that overpowering must have you-now suddenness. Also, because your bodies are adjusted unexpectedly, you can encounter absolutely new sensations.

Prepared to surrender standing sex a test drive? The following are the 5 positions our sex specialists suggest — each includes at any rate one, if not two, standing spouses.

1.   Use props to use your body weight.

Some customary sex positions are somewhat more instinctive, similar to missionary or doggy style. Sex standing up, in any case, can be all the more testing to pull off. Standing-up sex is incredible for challenging and brave sweethearts, yet the one thing that is absent from huge numbers of these upstanding positions is the part of dependability, which comes from a bed or level surface.

Stand eye to eye and have her spread her legs separated, so he can embed. A divider or a thin shower will turn into your best friend during standing sex in case you're battling to make it work, so she can set her feet against the divider for security while he pushes. Something to grab like a door handle, railing, or household item can likewise help influence your mate's body weight to assist her with feeling upheld. In addition, up close and personal considers all the more kissing and friendship.

2. Incline toward a wall for help.

Tallness can be an issue, and that those closer in stature may make some simpler memories pulling off this sex position. With standing sex, the penis is bound to sneak out, and the holding position might be a test to keep up for longer timeframes, yet not to stress: There are some workarounds so you can have that hot standing sex that you want. Couples can likewise have a go at staying strong with the man entering from behind. She can lean her pelvis back into him to get the ideal point or push ahead and curve her back if that feels good. This position can hit her G-spot, so he can pull back his pushes, make them more limited on the off chance that it feels great to her, or make them more profound if that is the thing that she needs.

3. Utilize your hands to make things much more sizzling.

Without a doubt, genital entrance alone can feel incredible during standing sex; however, if you battle to climax carefully from that; you can make this situation feel far superior by switching up push speed and contacting other delight focuses.

Known as standing doggy, take a stab at inclining at the midsection over a level surface like a work area and angling the back. Your spouse can hold your midriff and enter from behind. He can slow his developments and utilize shallow pushes joined with more profound pushes to give her G-recognize a little back rub. He can likewise reach over and animate her clitoris or her nipples.

4. Have a go at plunking down on a level surface for simple access.

This may sound irrational to having intercourse standing up, yet with one spouse standing and the other sitting on a high surface, you can have some vibe of great standing sex. It's a simple, fun, and unconstrained one that should be possible at home in for all intents and purposes any room, yet a kitchen or restroom counter, a table, or a clothes washer may help best because of stature. One mate can lift the other onto a high surface, which makes it simpler to get to. The situated spouse can lean their hands for help and fold their legs over the standing spouse. Since this doesn't happen in a bed, and maybe not even in the room, this has the quintessence of illegal sex, which can make this position vulgar.

5. Move to oral sex if things get abnormal.

It's not about genital penetration! You can have totally hot, feel-great sex standing up by utilizing your mouth. If you've attempted genital sex staying strong with no karma in arriving at a climax, alternate contribution oral sex to one another. While one spouse stands, the other can bow and perform oral sex on the other. Take a stab at folding one leg over your mate or setting a hand on his/or her head for direction.

6. Attempt shower sex, yet continue with alert.

A hot, hot shower is another incredible alternative for performing standing sex; however, it's critical to be aware of slipping or getting cleanser in your eyes.

Reverse sex should be possible in the shower while standing up or if one spouse is hanging over a stool, squeezing against a divider, or grasping a railing for added solidness. He additionally suggests utilizing grease since you can dry in the shower and water can wash away characteristic lube. Avoid utilizing cleanser as lubrication, as it very well may be aggravating, he cautions.

7. Reinforce your center.

Having an incredible sexual coexistence has the advantage of keeping you solid and fit. Standing sex, be that as it may, is considered by specialists to be marginally additionally burdening on your perseverance, particularly on the off chance that one spouse is holding up the other. This position can be awkward for extensive periods and can truly challenge a mate's arm quality on the off chance that the individual is holding the other spouse up. You likewise have the danger of falling.

Work on your center quality! You ought to do center activities if you need to have great sex, rising up to have the option to adjust and hold yourself up. This position initiates your lower center, back, hips, glutes, thighs, and then some, so reinforcing your center can assist you with supporting yourself and rock better.

8. Utilize standing sex as a type of foreplay.

On the off chance that you've experienced this rundown and still can't have a climax during standing sex, don't get baffled. Now and again, the infiltrating spouse discharges rapidly, and the accepting spouse may not arrive at the climax. You additionally might be utilized to sex on level surfaces and are more open to arriving at a climax that way.

Using standing sex as an energizing canapé and type of foreplay. At that point, couples can progress to a steadier situation for the primary course, where they're bound to climax.

The Best Sex Position During the Pregnancy

Discovering sex positions during pregnancy that are both agreeable and delight boosting may not be simple, yet we guarantee it's conceivable — regardless of what trimester you're in.

Knocking and pounding with a child on board may appear to be kinda alarming, particularly for first-time guardians; however, have confidence, research shows pregnancy sex is absolutely protected.

Truth be told, except if your primary care physician exhorts you in any case, don't hesitate to give a shot the same number of various pregnancy sex positions as you need throughout the following nine months. For example, in case you're in danger for an early conveyance, your primary care physician may suggest avoiding sex totally during the third trimester until around week 36, she adds.

The sex can feel astounding — like, considerably more astonishing than before you got pregnant. That is because, during incubation, your body's degrees of estrogen and progesterone rise. Those hormones heighten the bloodstream down there, which, thusly, ups vaginal grease and bosom affectability.

Be that as it may, even with every one of those pregnancy sex advantages, you may likewise encounter an adjustment in your solace level with specific positions. Since your body is changing, zones may get touchy to the point of torment; it is important to check in from week to week — and even every day — to understand what works, what feels better, and what doesn't.

In this way, while all positions are reasonable, you've most likely heard that it's perilous to lay on your back after week 20. That is halfway obvious — this can pack the vena cava, a significant vein that can affect flow all through your body, just as to your infant. Yet, before it gets to that point, it'll feel awkward. There's this generalization that you must have sex from the side or behind, yet you can have missionary sex if it doesn't keep going excessively long. Following five to 10 minutes, you may begin to feel odd, and you can simply move to your side by then.

The cervix cells are touchier during this time, as well, so they're bound to drain. You may see some spotting after sex — don't crack. All things being equal, if you spot under any conditions, consult your doctor regardless of whether you believe it's sex-related. Also, if sex doesn't feel incredible now, choose outercourse, oral sex, advanced infiltration, and anal sex — all safe for pregnant ladies.

Recall sex can incorporate toys, as well. Subbing your sex sesh with erotic touch and back rubs in case you're excessively worn out. It's an extraordinary method to interface and has closeness without there being tension on sex — particularly since some people get themselves route outside of the temperament. Take a stab at utilizing oils that bring an alternate aroma or even irregular articles that add to the vibe, similar to plumes.

In any case, in case you're in the mindset for some genuine under-the-sheets activity, let it all out! I believe it's so imperative to have intercourse during pregnancy since it keeps up closeness in love life. There's no motivation to be frightened of it. In addition, after you have the child, you'll be avoiding intercourse for around a month and a half, so get yours now.

1. Sex from behind

This position is frequently referred to by sex teachers as a well-known choice for a wide range of mates. Up down on the ground, this position keeps pressure off the tummy, permitting the pregnant spouse to remain more agreeable. Utilizing pads, covers, or towels to add comfort is an extraordinary thought.

Controlling the profundity of infiltration is likewise significant. Here and there, in that position with the ebb and flow of the back, [the pregnant spouse] can feel the penis hitting the cervix, which might be awkward. Perfect for the first and the start of the second trimesters. Before the second's over trimester, there's about an additional two pounds around your paunch. You might need to try not to adjust down on the ground during your most recent two months.

2. You on top

Move on board! This position is upheld by science, as well — at any rate, one Taiwanese examination discovered expanded sexual fulfillment for pregnant ladies who control infiltration by being on top of the spouse. Change for comfort by broadening your position or reclining to keep midsection weight from inclining you forward.

Great for the first and second trimesters. This position assists with hitting the correct spots in the vagina. Notwithstanding, during the third trimester, you might need to dodge profound entrance, particularly in case you're touchy down there and need to abstain from disturbing the cervix or incidental dying.

3. Spooning sex

Spooning is wonderful. It's a consoling position where the mate holds and generally infiltrates the pregnant spouse from behind while resting, both confronting endlessly from one another. However, if you're entering, consistently contact the clitoris as that is the place where the delight community seems to be. In later trimesters, it very well might be encouraging to hold the paunch. Always great for all trimesters, yet best during second and third as this position can help put less focus on the tummy.

4. Reverse cowgirl

Reverse cowgirl includes you, or the pregnant spouse, riding the other and is a decent choice in the first and second trimesters. Make certain to keep up the clitoral incitement in this position. Nonetheless, it tends to be testing later on when your paunch turns into a test. If this position is one of your top picks, you might have the option to change the weight by reclining and situating your arms behind you for help. Great for all trimesters, however during the second and third trimesters, you'll love this situation as it can shield your stomach from being packed — or contacted, in case you're touchy there.

6. Standing

On the off chance that under 20 weeks, a standing position works if your spouse is holding you around the midsection. Following 20 weeks, the stomach extension could cause more offset issues and trouble with position, which represents a danger of falling. The pregnant mate may put palms against a divider and lean in for steadiness. Be that as it may look for strong ground.

Experiment with this during the first and second trimesters; however, as your stomach develops, you may think that it's harder to hold this position. If it's pleasurable for your spouse, you could figure out how to join it close to the furthest limit of intercourse.

7. Skimming pregnant position

A pregnant individual may appreciate sex in the bath, where they can coast while giving or accepting joy. Lightness enables a midsection to resist gravity — a pleasant alternative when you're 8 months along.

Contingent upon the size of your tub, you will be unable to skim totally, so your spouse can support the experience. Have them lie under you for help and let their hands animate your delicate zones for joy. In the case of utilizing toys, make certain to utilize water-safe lube.

This works for all trimesters. Nonetheless, during the third trimester, when you're more delicate and charisma is low, this position is encouraging where climaxes don't need to be the end game. This can essentially be tied in with erotically thinking about one another.

8. Seated sex

Couples, all things considered, can appreciate situated intercourse, where the pregnant individual sits on a seat or on the edge of the bed, situating themselves over their mate. You can likewise prop yourself up with pads or lie on your back before pregnancy, or if agreeable. Their spouse would then be able to have simple access to fingers, toys, and mouths. Either by bowing before the pregnant individual, or grabbing a place to sit close to them and getting down to business. Perfect for all trimesters! This position is extraordinary for letting the body and gut rest.

5. Pregnant oral sex

Indeed, giving or getting oral sex is fine. It doesn't make a difference if you swallow in case you're giving oral sex to a spouse with a penis — it won't influence the child. Also, in case you're getting oral sex, it won't influence the infant, particularly in the last trimester.

Additionally, it's a wonderful option in contrast to penetrative sex in case you're only not available. Notwithstanding, if giving oral sex to a partner with a penis, know that during the primary trimester, you may have an elevated gag reflex because of morning affliction.

Good for all trimesters, in any event, when you're not pregnant. While clitoral incitement is one of the more solid ways to climax, not all sex requires to end in a climax. Sex is about physical closeness if there's infiltration or climaxes or not.

6. Anal sex

Truly, anal sex is protected during pregnancy and can be performed with your spouse at your back or while spooning. Doggy style, or entering from behind, would be the best for anal sex during pregnancy. You can likewise do this while spooning as well.

It's ideal on the off chance that you attempt this position from the get-go, before pregnancy, to perceive how agreeable you are with anal sex.

Recommendations

- Go slow and plan with foreplay for in any event 10 to 15 minutes.
- Use lube, particularly during pregnancy.
- Wear a condom for additional insurance against microorganisms and STIs.

Trimester: This position works for all trimesters. Notwithstanding, you'll need to be very cautious. Try not to move fingers, toys, tongue, or penis from butt to vagina. Doing so can spread microorganisms to the vagina, which could muddle pregnancy.

7. Next to each other sex

It's like spooning, aside from you're confronting one another. For any pregnant individual, positions on their side will feel good, and they can prop up their paunches with additional cushions or a moved-up towel. These side positions can be utilized for penetrative sex with hands and toys, just as for both giving and getting oral sex.

This means you can pivot and attempt 69 if that is something you like. Good for all trimester, best for third as it takes into consideration you or your pregnant spouse to lay on your sides without squeezing the stomach — or on one another!

CHAPTER 3:

Anal and Oral sex

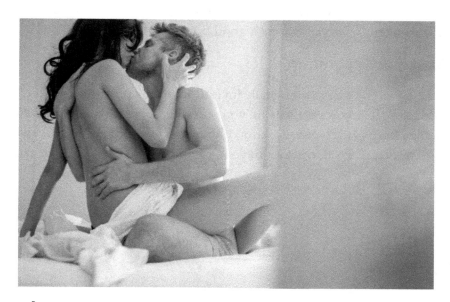

A nal sex is somewhat of a no-no subject, regardless of the way that it's an undeniably famous sexual behavior. As more couples investigate this kind of sex, understanding the dangers, rewards, and legitimate system is significant.

As indicated by the Centers for Disease Control (CDC), anal sex is principally developing in fame with couples below the age of 45. You may consider anal sex butt-centric entrance with a penis; however, you have a couple of more choices. Anal sex can likewise be performed with fingers or the tongue. Sex toys, such as butt plugs, dildos, and vibrators, are utilized as well.

Anybody can appreciate anal sex, regardless of whether they are a man, lady, gay, cross-sexual, or straight, and whether they are giving or getting it. Albeit numerous gay men appreciate it, some prefer not having penetrative anal sex. It is dependent upon you to choose what you need to try different things with and to discover what you appreciate.

Like any sexual behavior, anal sex isn't innately dangerous. It just requires all the more arranging, prep, and correspondence than some different types of sexual behavior. Well-being during sex should be the first concern; however, having a good time is positively significant.

Anal Sex Technique

At the point when you initially investigate the anal zone, it can feel odd, so before you start, ensure you and your spouse have discussed it and are both glad to give it a shot. On the off chance that you discover you don't care for it, disclose to your spouse that anal sex isn't for you.

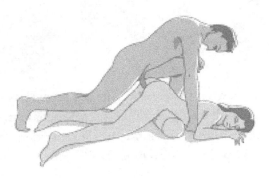

If you choose to have penetrative anal sex, start gradually with contacting and stroking to become accustomed to the thought and ensure you are loose. This is significant because there is a muscle in the rear-end (the sphincter) that should be loose to permit penetration to be enjoyable. On the off chance that you are giving anal sex, use a lot of grease and start by infiltrating only a little and afterward pulling out totally. At the point when your mate is prepared, enter somewhat further and afterward pull out once more. Proceed with this until you are completely in. Ensure you tune in to your spouse and see how they feel – be set up to stop whenever if they are awkward or in painfulness.

Anal sex can feel invigorating and pleasurable for both the individual giving and getting — yet it can likewise require a long time to become acclimated to how it feels. On the off chance that it doesn't go consummately, the first occasion when you can generally attempt again when you're both in the disposition. Recollect that you can interrupt or stop at whatever point you need. Because you have begun something doesn't mean you have to proceed.

Numerous men have sensitive spots in their prostate just as their butt, and they regularly appreciate having these animated. The prostate is between the bladder and the penis and can be animated with a finger or sex toy in the butt. Be that as it may, there are loads of veins in and around the prostate, and it can get wounded whenever took care of in general, so treat it delicately and use heaps of lube.

For some individuals, anal sex is a pleasurable piece of their sexual coexistence. Be that as it may, regardless of whether you are a man or a lady, penetrative anal sex can be awkward or even excruciating whenever surged, particularly if it's your first time.

Fortunately, there are things you can do to diminish any painfulness. These include making sure you are loose, going gradually, utilizing loads of water-based oil, and stirring your way up to the entrance with the penis with more modest items, such as fingers or sex toys.

Consistent correspondence is the ideal approach to ensure you both appreciate anal sex. If whenever you feel it is too awkward or difficult, at that point, you should stop right away.

Anal sex can be an extraordinary method to play around with your spouse. You simply need to give this new sexual experience a touch of arranging and readiness. However long you two are on the same wavelength about what you'd prefer to do and how you can partake in this experience together.

How might I make anal sex more secure?

- Use condoms to help ensure you prevent STIs when you have penetrative anal sex.
- Utilize a water-based ointment, which is accessible from drug stores. Oil-based oils (for example, cream and lotion) can make latex condoms break or fizzle.
- Get tips on utilizing condoms appropriately.
- Male and female couples should utilize another condom if they have vaginal sex straight after anal sex. This is to try not to move microbes from the butt to the vagina, which may prompt a urinary disease.

1. Talk with your spouse

Anal sex shouldn't be an unexpected solicitation mid-sex, as that'd be a significant infringement of trust and assent. In case you're keen on hard anal sex, discuss it with your mate. Come out to discuss it, and let them know you're interested.

On the off chance that the inclination is common, experience is standing by. If one of you chooses that anal sex simply isn't for you, that is alright. There are loads of alternatives for spicing things up in the room without adding anal sex.

2. Convey straightforwardly

Sorting out some way to do anal sex with your spouse starts with correspondence. Discussion about it first. Similarly, as with a wide range of sexual behavior, anal sex is something that should be talked about already. Impart your feelings of trepidation and desires with your spouse, and ensure that you are both in the same spot about things like speed, profundity, and so forth. Trust me, this is one region in which you don't need any amazements.

3. Think about a douche

Concerned that doing the filthy will be dirty? It's conceivable. On the off chance that you need things spotless down there, you can utilize a purification to clean the lower half of your rectum after a solid discharge; however, it's a bit much. You can discover these items, all things considered, at medication stores and drug stores.

4. Cut your nails

Diminish your danger of cutting or scratching your spouse by managing your nails. Long nails may tear the slight, sensitive tissue of the butt, which could prompt dying. It likewise expands the danger of spreading microscopic organisms that could cause diseases.

Make certain to wash your hands well and scour under your nails after anal sex, as well, particularly before embeddings them into the vagina or mouth.

5. Wear a condom or dental dam

Individuals who have anal sex have a higher risk of sharing STIs, however, utilizing a condom or dental dam diminishes that hazard. If you need to move from the butt to the vagina, make certain to utilize another condom. In case you're not utilizing a condom, wash the penis — or a toy in case you're utilizing that — a long time before embeddings it into the vagina.

6. Get in position

Numerous individuals discover lying on their stomachs with their mate behind them functions admirably for anal sex. Missionary can work, as well, as long as you change the purpose of the passage. Doggy style is additionally a simple position. The open spouse can gradually back up onto the insertive spouse to control profundity and movement.

7. Unwind your body and mind

The exact opposite thing you need to be before endeavoring anal entrance (or anal incitement) is tense. In case you're reluctant, anxious, or not into it, nobody will get off, and what's the purpose of that? If this is your first time attempting anal sex, invest some energy unwinding — clean up, request that your spouse give you an erotic back rub, hell, you can even contemplate. To get ready for anal sex, you can likewise zero in on explicitly loosening up the muscles of your anal sphincter. To perceive what that feels like, fix your butt muscles — sort of like a kegel for the opposite end — and afterward discharge.

8. Set up Boundaries

All through the experience, you must focus on what you are feeling and impart this to your mate. If something feels awkward or agonizing, let them know. You may decide to set up a protected word to tell your spouse you're not happy with pushing ahead or that you need to move a little slower.

9. Lather up

Numerous ladies' dread of first-time anal sex comes from a dread of what goes on back there (normally) and how that will play into the activity. To purify yourself (in a real sense) of such mental barricades, take a pleasant, hot shower first.

10. Participate in a lot of foreplay

Probably the ideal approach to slide into anal play is to ensure you're incredibly stirred previously. The main slip-up individuals make is surging. Start with foreplay, vaginal sex, whatever turns you on. (Being a couple of climaxes profound before you attempt any anal entrance helps.) The more excited you are, the more loosened up your sphincter muscle will be, and that will make for a more sultry and simpler experience.

11. Lube is an unquestionable requirement

For comfort, you'll have to give your own grease — and a lot of it. Search for a water-based choice, as it won't separate the condom you're wearing. Keep a wash material, or infant wipes convenient to tidy up from abundance lube. In contrast to the vagina, the rear-end doesn't deliver its own grease. The more lube you use, the more enjoyable and charming anal sex can be. Remember to ensure you are utilizing a condom-safe, water or silicone-based grease (oil-based oils aren't viable with condoms). Try not to be hesitant to reapply as often as possible. More lube rises to better anal sex consistently.

12. Go moderate and check in with your mate often

Try not to hop into anal sex cold. Give yourself 10 to 15 minutes of foreplay to heat up. This encourages you — and the anal sphincter — to unwind, which can make the experience more agreeable.

Take things gradually, use a lot of oil, and stop if it turns out to be excessively excruciating. Try not to plan to have full penis entrance your first go-round.

Take a stab at utilizing a finger, and afterward, move up to a few fingers. A toy may be a decent alternative, as well, as you develop more OK with the sensation. After the first run-through or two, you and your spouse will probably find that the joy bests any underlying inconveniences.

13. Expect the correct position

For first-time anal sex, the collector (otherwise known as whichever spouse is being infiltrated) should be the one to control the profundity and speed of entrance.

The ideal situation to permit you to do that is you on top, which gives you full control of exactly how quick and profound you go.

14. Move slowly

Regardless of how much lube you use, your secondary passage isn't a water slide. First-time anal sex should be moved toward getting into a truly hot bath. First, you try things out during foreplay, permitting your mate to delicately rub around the opening with their finger before exploring different avenues regarding really embeddings anything. Regardless of whether you're utilizing a penis, a finger, or a toy, start gradually with simply the tip before embeddings anything any more profound.

15. Attempt a toy

Utilizing a little dildo or anal fitting can be an incredible method to slide into things. The key here is to be delicate and impart. On the off chance that anytime things get excessively awkward, shout out.

16. You must not cross-fertilize

Regardless of whether it's a finger, a toy, or a penis, try never to go from butt to vagina — it's a UTI already in the works. On the off chance that you need to change to vaginal incitement after anal play, bounce in the shower to prop the activity up or keep a tub of child wipes on your end table to disinfect in the middle.

17. Make sure to relax

In those initial couple of seconds of penetration, the weight will generally reason ladies to hold their breath. This outcome is the prompt fixing of those muscles, which will just prompt torment. Take profound, even breaths and spotlight on loosening up your whole body and delivering all pressure. It might feel like you need to go to the washroom from the start, however, go with it.

18. Say it if there is pain

First-time anal play will be brimming with new sensations, some peculiar, some astonishing. What you shouldn't feel is torment. If anytime during the activity, entrance becomes difficult, let your spouse know right away. You might need to add more lube, slow things down, or give it a rest for some time and change to different sorts of incitement.

19. Utilize a condom

Because there's no danger of getting pregnant doesn't mean you can skirt the condom — they're the best way to forestall explicitly sent contaminations. Simply don't go from anal to vaginal infiltration with a similar condom as that can spread diseases. Jettison the condom and put on another one preceding entering the vagina.

20. Remember vaginal incitement

There are many mutual sensitive spots between the dividers of the vagina and the rear-end, so invigorating the vagina at the same time can be very pleasurable. If you feel good, embed something (maybe a finger or a vibrator) into your vagina while you are participating in anal play.

21. Change it up

As you get more alright with anal sex with a spouse you trust, you can investigate various positions. Spooning is another extraordinary pick for secondary passage learners. Its position gives you shared control of your developments and adds an additional dash of closeness, which may enable you to unwind too. Doggy-style position permits your spouse simple passage yet, in addition, places them in full control, which probably won't be the best for your first time. If you feel torment anytime, have your mate back off, stop, or switch positions.

22. Try not to worry about it

If you are pondering when is the correct opportunity to participate in first-time anal sex, recall that there's no set-in-stone answer. For certain ladies, anal sex is off-limits, and for others, it's a chance. Whichever way is a-OK.

23. Acknowledge that there will probably be some crap included

This is, essentially, a truth of anal sex. Regardless of whether you do wash or utilize a bowel purge in advance. On the off chance that the possibility of crap jumping on you makes you awkward, anal sex may not be the correct choice for you.

24. Tidy up thereafter or before you do whatever else

Although your rear-end and rectum are cleaner than you may suspect, minute fecal issues will consistently be available. You can lessen your danger of disease by changing condoms and washing them admirably. You ought to never go from butt to vagina or mouth without tidying up first.

Anal Sex for Deep Orgasm

Anal sex can prompt climax, yet that doesn't need to be the planned result. Anal sex can simply be a great method to play. For certain individuals, the rear-end is an erogenous zone. So, even only a little play can be a turn-on. The rear-end is additionally brimming with touchy sensitive spots, so it's exceptionally open to sexual incitement. For the insertive spouse, the snugness around the penis can be satisfying also.

Anal sex additionally invigorates the prostate organ in men, which can upgrade a man's climax. For ladies, clitoral incitement might be important during anal sex to arrive at the peak, yet only one out of every odd lady will arrive at climax along these lines. Oral or vaginal sex might be important to arrive at the peak.

An anal orgasm is the aftereffect of sexual incitement of the nerves in and around the rear-end. The rear-end is [packed] with nerves, particularly the unbelievably erogenous pudendal nerve associated with the clitoris. The pudendal nerve conveys sensation to and from your perineum, arriving at your vagina, vulva, and rear-end, as well.

What does this sort of climax feel like? A few ladies portray it as being like a clitoral climax—a beat of pleasurable compressions, however, this time around the anal sphincter. Others may feel even more a "spreading wave" of supplication. Some ladies may hit this high note during penetrative anal sex with their spouse's penis, while others arrive through lighter contacting or utilizing toys. Like some other sort of climax, there's no "correct" approach to do it, and each lady has her own method relying upon what feels bravo body and her own solace level.

All things considered, the best approach to begin is to explore. Pleasurable anal play can occur with a butt-centric vibrator, attachment or globules, a penis or dildo, finger play, analingus, truly anything.

Like any sort of sex meeting, you'll need to get things moving with sufficient measures of foreplay, for example, contacting, kissing, and vaginal and clitoral incitement. From that point, slide into it. Go slowly, utilize your hands, help your mate unwind, and ensure that it is no joke.

Whenever you're loose and prepared, start with a tongue or finger to tenderly invigorate the territory of the rear-end. At the point when you're stirred, attempt to ease one finger or tip of an attachment inside. The muscles will open up normally so the attachment or finger can head inside. On the off chance that you need to compel it, you're not prepared.

From that point, you can have a go at something greater — an attachment, lash on dildo, or penis, for instance. On the off chance that the fitting or finger effectively slide all through the rear-end without inconvenience, you might need to move into penetrative sex. On the off chance that you pick a toy, one that is marginally more than your finger, no more extensive than two fingers, non-finished, and made of an adaptable material.

As you get more into it, your anal region may begin feeling excessively pleasurable sensations, even a development of weight that segues into constriction-like waves. On the off chance that what you experience isn't exactly the delivery you regularly feel when you climax, it should even now feel better.

In case you're encountering astounding sensations, yet you're not exactly arriving at peak yet you continue attempting, take a full breath — and take having a climax off the table. Weight, stress, and uneasiness are the greatest blockers of climax. Have a go at remaining at the time when you investigate the vibes of anal play. Likewise, with any sort of climax, don't let the end game become the entire game.

Oral Sex

Oral sex, also known as blow jobs, rimming, or going down, is the stimulation of a partner's private parts with the mouth, tongue, or lips. Oral sex could be fellatio (licking or sucking the penis), cunnilingus (licking or sucking the clitoris, vagina, or vulva), or anilingus (licking or sucking the anus).

Oral sex is also known as blow jobs, rimming, or going down. In any case, what's the ideal approach to do it? Regardless of whether you are considering having oral sex unexpectedly or simply need some more data — read on for tips on how to appreciate safe oral sex. Oral sex includes utilizing your mouth or tongue to animate your spouse's privates or butt.

Numerous individuals appreciate oral sex as a component of their sexual coexistence; however, it is an extremely close-to-home thing, and not every person likes it or decides to do it. Various individuals like to give or get oral sex in various manners. There is an entire assortment of approaches to lick, suck, and animate somebody. You may choose not to involve in oral sex by any means, or you may appreciate exploring different avenues regarding your mate to discover what gives you both joy.

It is critical to converse with your spouse so you can comprehend what the both of you appreciate and what you would like to evade. It can require a long time to work out what causes somebody to feel great. The best activity is to continue speaking with your spouse. Request that they mention to you what feels decent and let them know when you appreciate something.

In case you're upbeat and happy with somebody, oral sex can be an extraordinary method to get truly nearer and realize what turns each other on. On the off chance that you discover you detest something, you can stop whenever you need it, and the equivalent is valid for your spouse.

How would you give a man oral sex?

A man's penis needn't be erect for you to begin oral sex (a sensual caress); however, you might need to utilize your hand to stimulate him first. On the off chance that you hold his penis during oral sex, you can control how profound it goes into your mouth. You can move your hand, permitting the penis to go as far into your mouth as you are alright with.

A man's penis is profoundly touchy, so be delicate from the outset and gradually work up to a quicker movement. You can attempt distinctive tongue, mouth, and head developments to perceive what works best; however, never utilize your teeth except if inquired.

At the point when you give a man oral sex, you can stop whenever and it's dependent upon you to choose if you need to allow him to discharge (or cum) into your mouth. Obviously, if he's wearing a condom, this isn't an issue, and it implies you will both be secured against explicitly sent contaminations (STIs).

How would you give a lady oral sex?

Before you start giving a lady oral sex, she may appreciate it on the off chance that you invest some energy kissing and contacting her upper thighs and the territory around her vagina first to assist her with getting stirred.

The entire genital territory is delicate, yet for most ladies, the clitoris (with its 8,000 sensitive spots) is the most touchy part. Tenderly, part the external lips of the vagina and search for the vaginal opening and the hooded clitoris simply above it.

Start off delicately, utilizing a casual tongue to make sluggish developments and work up to quicker developments with a firmer tongue. You can analyze moving your tongue in various manners and attempt various rhythms — following your mate to discover what she appreciates most.

How would you give oral-anal sex (rimming)?

Performing oral sex on your spouse's rear-end (otherwise called rimming) can be essential for any sexual love story, regardless of whether gay, indiscriminate, or straight. If you are worried about cleanliness, request that your spouse wash first. You could likewise wash together as a feature of foreplay.

Before you start, your mate may like it if you tenderly kiss and contact the zone around the butt, including the perineum (the zone of skin between the privates and the rear-end). You would then be able to zero in on the rear-end, surrounding your tongue around the external region lastly, embeddings your tongue. Make sure to tune in to your spouse and do what they appreciate, regardless of whether that is licking, sucking, or delicately examining.

If you are giving oral sex to a lady, don't move from the butt to the vagina as this can move microorganisms and cause contamination.

How to ensure a more secure oral sex?

- When oral sex is on a male partner, a condom may be utilized to lessen the danger of contracting sexually transmitted infections. Attempt a seasoned one if you don't care for the flavor of ordinary condoms.
- When the oral sex is on a female partner, utilize a dam. The same is applicable for anilingus. A dam is a little, tiny square of plastic or latex that goes about as an obstruction between the mouth and anus or vagina for forestalling spreading sexually transmitted infections.
- You can get dams and condoms at health clinics on the web, or drug stores may also arrange to help you deliver them.

CHAPTER 4:

Dirty talk

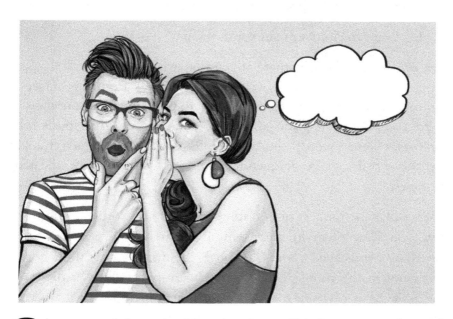

S ince one of the main things in a love affair is correspondence, it possibly bodes well that when things get hot and weighty, you should keep on having an exchange. Truly, I'm proposing the dirty talk, and indeed, on the off chance that you haven't checked it out during sex or foreplay, now is the ideal time. It's, in reality, not so frightening.

While there are a lot of incredible articles out there about how to speak profanely to your spouse, there aren't sufficient out there regarding why you ought to do it. However, those pieces appear to fail to remember that when you carry dirty talking with the general mish-mash, it isn't just about your spouse and their requirements; it's similarly about what you appreciate, as well, and a ton of us truly love to speak profanely. It feels great to allow everything to out.

How It Can Help with Sex Life

Regardless of whether you decide to speak profanely in bed, through sexting, or like to enjoy classic telephone sex, dirty talk is certainly something everybody should attempt. Here are eight hot reasons why.

1. You can discover your comfortability

The explanation for why there are endless articles about how to speak profanely is because it very well may be dubious from the outset. It can cause a few people to feel powerless to put themselves out there in quite a vocal manner, and afterward, there are the individuals who can't state certain words, similar to "pussy," or "dick," which, frankly, are the words you're frequently going for when you're speaking profanely.

There's likewise the test of defeating how you see words in reality and how you view them in the room. It's absolutely acceptable to be turned by words like "whore," although you may discover them hostile when not in the room. You're assuming responsibility for the word and utilizing it on your standing, and that can be trying for certain ladies. However, now and again, a test encourages you to characterize what you're OK with — on your own terms.

2. It helps your partner know what you want

Except if you're dating a mystical human, your mate can't guess what you might be thinking. At the point when you express what feels better, what needs some work, or that your clitoris is only somewhat higher, and you'd truly love it if your spouse could concentrate all their energy there; at that point, you both benefits.

When you can both say what you like and how you like it, you're not very far away from saying how it affects you. From that point, the dirty talk will simply stream — it will take practice, however, obviously.

3. It gets you flowing

Along these lines, possibly your form of speaking profanely right currently is telling your spouse that you're going to come. That is typically one part of dirty talk that individuals can handle, yet consider how hot it is to simply let free and uncover all the things you keep in your mind during sex.

Before you know it, you've gone from hollering, "I'm coming! I'm coming!" to something about how you will appear at your mate's work, lock them in their office, and give them the kind of mid-day break that you've both consistently needed. At that time, you've made a dream and a situation that you can hold returning to and can expand upon. Perhaps you'll even wind up receiving your own adaptation of Fifty Shades of Gray in return — you never know!

4. It's a great form of foreplay

As any specialist or sex advisor will let you know, foreplay is a critical piece of sex, particularly for ladies. It makes ladies far longer to get stirred than men, which is why they don't climax as fast as men do. As far as we might be concerned, foreplay is fundamental.

On the off chance that you can begin with some dirty talk; at that point, you'll be tempting each other in manners that are similarly as significant as actual foreplay. Quick ones are fun, yet on the off chance that you have the opportunity to take as much time as is needed, at that point, do it. Put aside an entire 20 minutes of simply speaking profanely to one another before you even take off your garments and contact one another. You'll see the distinction it makes.

5. It's a great surprise for you

It's consistently pleasant when you can even now astonish yourself, right? Also, the thing is, the point at which you drive yourself to accomplish something that you've never done, you could very well acknowledge it was made for you. Speaking graphically about how you need to be contacted and how you will contact your spouse may reform your sexual coexistence — yet you'll actually discover except if you check it out.

6.   ...and for your spouse

There are a lot of approaches to zest things up in your drawn-out love life when things are feeling somewhat old. On the off chance that your sexual coexistence has become the stuff of missionary just before bed, in that moment, speaking profanely to your spouse is a simple method to change it up a piece.

Odds are the grimy things you've been thinking, yet haven't said for all to hear yet, will really astonish them. You can murmur in your spouse's ear, ensuring your lips just somewhat brush their ear cartilage. From that point, contingent upon their reaction, you can proceed, or let them dominate and mention to you their opinion, as well.

7.   Your sex would be better

In case you're talking truly, straightforwardly, and graphically about what you need to escape each sexual experience, in what manner can it not prompt better sex? With correspondence and so much dirty talk, there are no insider facts — and neither you nor your spouse is compelled to attempt to sort out what that groan or outward appearance truly implies. Sex shouldn't be a puzzle.

8.   The fun is immense

You may believe that you must be totally genuine when you're speaking profanely, yet you don't. A ton of times, individuals fail to remember that in addition to the fact that sex is fun — it tends to be entertaining, as well. If you can slacken up enough to make some great memories, chuckle about it, and unwind; you'll be stunned by what kind of good time you can have.

Fun with Sex Toys

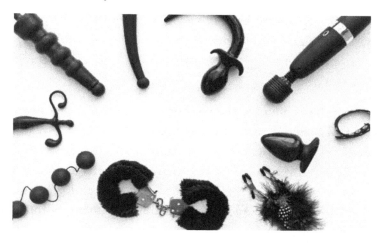

With regards to playing with your mate, it's an ideal opportunity to get into the mood for sex. Or then again, cuffs! Or then again, to fiddle with massage oils, twofold dildos, and vibrators that are extremely popular in these times. Name the coupled needing, and the sex toy goddesses have probably cooked up an approach to satisfy it. We've developed far past the times of the rabbit standard. Nowadays, twofold dildos are looking pretty damn smooth. Vibrators pack remarkably non-double energy, and their frequently erogenous zone-satisfying plans can consistently progress with you from solo masturbation to sex with your spouse. Also, concerning old-fashioned penis rings? They comfort the vaginal waterway. They crush the peen. They vibrate. They gleam. Stirring up your coupled sexual coexistence can be as simple and reasonable as purchasing a blindfold or as long-game vital as putting resources into a butt plug preparing unit (for the Virgos out there; we see you). We've generally advocated vibrators as apparatuses for a self-sufficient climax, yet they actually can likewise be a lighting bar into foreplay and sex with your spouse(s), regardless of whether you're in a submitted love story or simply a horny tumbleweed on a delight twisting, each spouse play toy can show you more your necessities. Consider it another method of opening up your connections.

1. Dildos

While they may appear to be practically less interesting in contrast with all the vibrating, innovative, activity stuffed toys accessible now, dildos are still an exemplary toy that a lot of ladies and considerably more men are super into.

In case you're searching for the passion of entrance that is nearest to a genuine penis, dildos are the best approach. They arrive in an assortment of shapes, lengths, and widths, so consider when you're shopping (a few ladies may find that marginally bent ones are better at getting them off since they'll give your clit and G-spot more straightforward activity), and consider utilizing them both vaginally and anally.

2. Penis Rings

Penis rings were initially made to give people with penises a more extended, more full erection since they pack the veins and make the penis more delicate. Presently, there are vibrating penis rings, which offer a similar impact while giving a buzzy sensation to the wearer and the spouse being infiltrated. They're additionally an extraordinary method to transform dildos into vibrating dildos for lash on sex

3. Butt Plugs

Consider butt plugs first experience with anal play. Anal toys are famous with ladies although they have no prostate or nerves to legitimately cause climax inside the rear-end; they can be a tremendous mental turn-on. In case you're a novice, start with a shower and get spotless heretofore, and afterward, have your mate animate you with his fingers — or tongue, if he's gutsy — before embeddings a fitting, vibrator, or dots. Use latex gloves or condoms on fingers for neatness and anal lube for solace and skim.

4. Nipple Clamps

Connecting these folks to your pinches harms — however it should. Such a large amount of BDSM play is about the sort of painfulness that can be a hot sensation for some individuals, if for reasons unknown other than the way that it's so unique concerning what we feel on a regular premise. Numerous clips accompany extravagant highlights like movable weight, a vibrating choice, and waterproof covering; however, clothespins can be similarly as compelling if you would prefer not to purchase genuine ones.

5. Prostate Toys

Worked for individuals with prostates (male, generally), these toys can give direct sensation to the prostate — some of them vibrate, while others don't. They're a thin, bent toy that is like G-spot toys. They give direct sensation to the prostate and are an incredible choice for individuals who need to investigate prostate play yet don't have any desire to utilize their hands.

6. Vibrators

These should be your go-to sex toy for solo and couple's play. It is recommended that ladies have an assortment of vibrators — various shapes, sizes, and kinds of triggers to coordinate their disposition and whatever sensation they're searching for at that point. At times you may need a major, vibrating dildo that you can push at your own rhythm, and on different occasions, you should utilize a vibrating butt plug. Try not to stress that utilizing a vibrator consistently will overstimulate your clit or play with your capacity to accompany a classic penis — that is a legend.

7. Cuffs

Cuffs are more about the psychological and passionate turn-on than the actual sensation. It tends to be very exciting to examine the scene you'll set up and get the important assent. It's a spectacular imagination play and is increasing greater fame as a result of ongoing presentation and standardization in the media. Simply be cautious — in case you're going for a real detainee dream that includes genuine metal handcuffs, they can hurt.

8. Clitoral Massagers

For ladies who make some extreme memories coming from other sex toys (or spouses, even), a vibrator that centers absolutely around invigorating the most delicate portion of your vagina could be the silver projectile. Distressingly, men don't invest enough energy in clitoral play, and ladies stay quiet about their clitoral necessities. Utilize your clitoral massager while being pushed; use it a short time later when you're swollen and he's nodded off; let the person in question see you utilizing it, so it turns into a couple's action

9. Anal Beads

Marginally not quite the same as butt connects that they embed each individual dab in turn, as opposed to easily and progressively like an attachment, butt-centric dabs furnish a pop inclination with each bigger size that goes in. And keeping in mind that such an anal toy and play will help prep you for genuine anal sex, butt attachments may be a touch more like how that will feel.

Sexual Fantasies

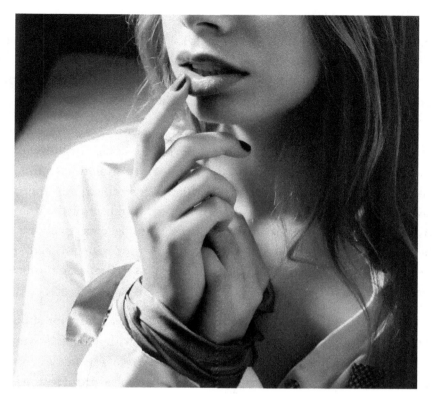

An erotic fantasy or sexual fantasy is a psychological picture or example of thinking that arouses an individual's sexuality and can make or improve sexual arousal. A sexual imagination can be made by the individual's creative mind or memory and might be set off self-sufficiently or by outside incitement; for example, sensual writing or erotic entertainment, an actual article, or sexual appreciation for someone else. Anything that may offer ascent to a sexual excitement may likewise deliver a sexual imagination, and sexual excitement may thusly offer ascent to imaginations.

Sexual fantasies exist in every single diverse size and form. For a few, it can mean essentially bringing a bunny vibrator into the room for some extra clitoral incitement. For other people, it could mean hanging a roof sex swing, snatching a few cuffs, making sure about a blindfold, and purchasing calfskin undergarments. Thus, no doubt, there's somewhat of a range.

In any case, paying little heed to what you might be keen on, investigating sexual imaginations are an incredible way not exclusively to spice up things in the room in the manner that makes you happy, yet it can remove the dullness from your ordinary everyday.

Yet, recall, regardless of how explicit your sexual imagination is, each sexual demonstration all through the room should begin with a discussion — and that is correct; this implies you should have the sex talk with your spouse consistently. What this resembles: For one, you have to build up a protected word. This word would simply be utilized to transfer to your spouse that the scene is going excessively far or there's a limit being crossed. You, as well as your mate, should stop promptly once a protected word is raised. This guarantees protected consensual sex.

The second thing you can do is simple: Just discuss with your spouse. Since you're jumping into a new sexual area with whatever you're trying, here are a few inquiries you should present in advance to ensure you're checking in with your spouse and their pleasure. How will I know whether you're having some good times? By what method will I know when I have to accomplish something other than what's expected? What sort of disposition or passion would we like to have while we play?

1. Multi-mate sex

Multi-spouse sex includes sex with more than one person of different or the same sexes. Sex with three spouses might be known as a threesome, and more partners might be known as an orgy. A recent report distributed in Archives of Sexual Behavior of Canadian college students uncovered that 64% of them fantasized about multi-mate sex.

Another examination distributed in Personality and Individual Differences, including 788 British grown-ups, found that men explicitly may fantasize more about multi-spouse sex. Male members of the examination were bound to fantasize about sex with different individuals and with mysterious spouses. Then, ladies' imaginations were bound to incorporate same-sex spouses and famous individuals.

2. Predominant or harsh sex

Harsh sex is a sexual demonstration that is forceful, bestial, and maybe fairly vicious. It is regularly portrayed as more enthusiastic than different sorts of sex; however, it can likewise be related to unfortunate damaging sex. However, harshness isn't intrinsically risky or oppressive.

BDSM, which represents bondage, discipline/domination, submission/sadism, and masochism envelops a lot of unpleasant sex encounters. BDSM incorporates various kinks or activities — regularly thought to be atypical sexual practices. Prevailing or compliant sex regularly includes the consensual expecting and giving up of intensity between those included. It can include bondage, beating, and a whole range of different practices and romantic snares.

A few people are excited by light limitation, others by actual extreme torment. Mental roleplay — like that between an educator and understudy or a chief and worker — may likewise be viewed as BDSM as it includes a trade of intensity.

3. Voyeurism or exhibitionism

Voyeurism is excitement brought about by viewing a clueless individual or individuals occupied with a private close or sexual act. A little 1991 examination discovered 54% of men have voyeuristic imaginations.

Exhibitionism is the opposite of voyeurism; it is the demonstration of getting stimulated by others consensually watching you have intercourse or by uncovering portions of your body to clueless members. Both of these crimps can be viewed as risky if one can't control their inclinations if the imagination causes passionate misery, or if lawful issues emerge.

You likely won't have the option to follow up on this sexual imagination. In the US and numerous different nations, it is unlawful to watch or tape anybody having intercourse without their assent. Also, public nakedness is unlawful in the greater part of the US, although the meaning of bareness may fluctuate by state.

4.   Open sex or an irregular place

Sex out in the open is another mainstream imagination that may fall under exhibitionism. In Lehmiller's equivalent overview, he discovered 81% of men and 84% of ladies were excited by a public sex imagination. Note that following up on this imagination is regularly illicit. Although real rules differ by region — for example, public bareness is legitimate in regions like Denver where individuals of all genders can go topless — sex acts in broad daylight are unlawful in each of the 50 states.

5.   Roleplay and cosplay

Notwithstanding their comparative names, these two fantasies are different. Roleplay is the suspicion of another personality. During a sexual demonstration, pretend can be a piece of a significant number of the above crimps. For instance, it can assist individuals with playing out imaginations of irregular intensity characteristics or as outsiders. Cosplay is the demonstration of dressing up like some other person or thing, regularly from a book, film, or computer game. It isn't inalienably sexual; however, a few people appreciate imitating a character during sex.

Tragically, there has not been a lot of examination done on the subject of these fantasies. An issue in the International Journal of Roleplaying proposes this is because sexologists believe it to be an "immaterial factor of foreplay and thusly, isn't expressly remembered for research polls."

6. Romantic sex

Romantic or amorous sex is unique concerning numerous imaginations because there is no predetermined definition — what is passionate for one individual may vary for another.

In principle, any sort of sex can be passionate. Romantic sex is a sexual love affair wherein there's a passionate and sensual association. It very well may be long and moderate and sexy; it very well may be tantric sex, it might, you be able to know, have some BDSM associated with it.

Tantric sex, for instance, is moderate and doesn't focus its ultimate objective on climax. All things being equal, its objective is to zero in on the whole sexual experience and any sensations it raises.

It was reported that sexual imaginations are more famous among more youthful respondents of his study. He likewise discovered 91% of straight men, 88% of straight ladies, and 87% of gay and swinger people fantasize about their present spouse — making spouses the most widely recognized individual respondents fantasized about.

7. Homoeroticism and gender-bending

Sex bowing is the point at which an individual defies cultural desires for their sex. Current American instances of it date back to 1920s vaudeville and can be connected to modern shows. Individuals of all sexual directions can rehearse this fantasy. Note that this is not the same as transgenderism, which is the point at which somebody has a sexual orientation character or sex articulation that varies from their relegated sex upon entering the world.

Homoeroticism is an imagination that includes sexual acts with individuals of a similar sex. It tends to be — and is frequently — experienced by individuals who recognize as heterosexual, not simply gay or eccentric.

Further, sexual longing isn't either circumstance nor does it characterizes your sexual personality. For instance, a hetero cisgender lady who is in an explicitly satisfying love life with a cisgender man can at present have imaginations about other ladies.

Fox considers sexuality a range or a ringer bend. On one tail of the bend is totally straight, and on the other tail is in effect totally gay. A great many people fall someplace in the center. Individuals may recognize as straight; however, they can have a little sensation about envisioning, or in any event, connecting with sexual acts that are of the same sex. Some straight individuals do have intercourse with a similar sex individual occasionally.

How to Introduce Sexual Fantasies to your Partner

Evaluating sexual imaginations with your mate is energizing and exciting. Yet, before you start, there are significant parts of experimentation you ought to guarantee are set up for most extreme security and joy.

1. Set up assent

The main thing to build up when having intercourse with spouses is assent. It shows the spouse you regard and their body, and a sexual demonstration without assent is attacked. Assent is express, non-coercive authorization to participate in a specific demonstration, for this situation, one of a sexual sort. It tends to be renounced whenever. It is the most crucial part of solid sex.

Assent isn't only recognizing "no" as "no" — however, to a greater degree, a "yes" implies "yes." It appears as though consistently checking in with a mate all through a sexual encounter, asking expressly on the off chance that they like something before you do it, and discontinuing a demonstration if they request that you stop — regardless of whether they consented to it already

2. Talk about limits

To have the most secure conceivable experience, you should be straightforward about what it is you need and don't need. This can include setting a plan for how the sexual experience may go, including what is beyond reach, and establishing a protected word to state when you start to feel panicked, so your spouse realizes when to stop. The premise of these limits is assent, which can be surrendered whenever. It is imperative to get authorization before taking a stab at anything new, or regardless of whether it's something you do routinely.

3. Utilize legitimate security

To try not to transmit any STIs, guarantee you practice safe sex with a condom or other obstruction. Different types of contraception like an IUD or spermicide don't secure against STIs; educate your mate already if you might be conveying one.

4. Approach your spouse with deference

Sex is private and should just be experienced someplace and with somebody with who you have a sense of security. Comprehend that weakness must be grasped when having intercourse, and don't state or do whatever may cause your spouse to feel judged. Move slowly, particularly while attempting new things. Voice any worries or considerations you may have all through.

CHAPTER 5:

Tantric Sex

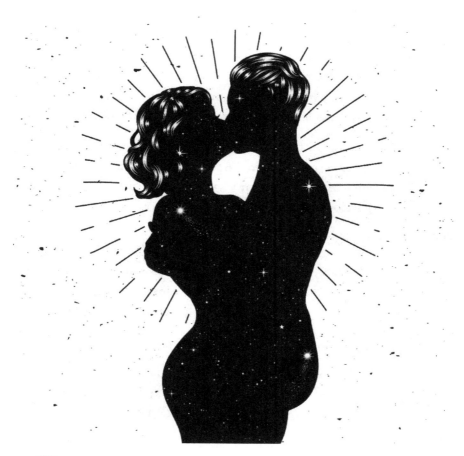

O n the off chance that you've wanted sex that is better, longer-enduring, and cozier — and let's face it, who isn't — it very well may be an ideal opportunity to attempt tantric sex. Tantric sex is an eased back down, striking, very hot method of engaging in sexual relations. Tantra is how you accomplish something;

it's the rule you apply. Thus, truly, you can do any movement — and any sex position — tantrically.

On the off chance that it astonishes you, you're in good company. Individuals have every one of these thoughts and confusions about tantra sex and what it looks like. Tantra really doesn't look that changed outwardly; it just feels diverse within because it's sex in addition to that internal association.

That implies you don't have to gain proficiency with an entirely different arrangement of sex aptitudes and additional setups. All things being equal, you will only have to apply a tantric flair to improve the positions you definitely know by easing back down, de-focusing the climax, keeping in touch, and zeroing in on profound adoring.

All things considered, a few positions loan themselves to tantric sex in a way that is better than others. Apologies, yet places that require accomplishments of wellness (for example, handcart, scissoring, and standing split) are best put something aside for some other time.

What Is Tantric Sex?

Tantric sex is an important sexual practice that is part of the profound antiquated way known as tantra. Tantra is a Sanskrit expression that means "weave." It alludes to weaving together or joining the manly and ladylike powers inside us all, paradise and earth, the human body with the religious, falling the polarities. The motivation behind tantra is to find a delighted association with all of life past the different ability to be self-aware. Holy or tantric sex is viewed as one entryway to that religious truth when we figure out how to tackle it.

The easiest clarification of tantric closeness is that it's tied in with bringing the fire of your sexual energy, enthusiasm, and wants into an arrangement with your heart, your soul, and a feeling of goodness in your life. At the point when these powers come into equilibrium and concordance, the flashes of relational wizardry truly begin flying, and sex becomes something recuperating, engaging, extraordinary, and significantly excellent.

Albeit frequently inseparable from sex, tantra is truly about association — regardless of whether that is with yourself or among you and a spouse. All things considered, the word itself — got from the old Sanskrit — signifies "web" or "to weave energy." By and by, tantra is about edification: to rise above both the sexual and profound planes by participating in profoundly thoughtful, unconstrained, and personal sex.

Tantric Sex Technique

1. Establish a holy region.

Get into the mindset is by consolidating ceremonies into sex. That can be anything, for example, setting up your space as a safe haven with candles, delicate music, and pillows. What's most significant is that you cause sex to feel exceptional. You need a feeling that sex is something significant and particular from regular day-to-day existence.

Intentionally disengage from the everyday world and enter the universe of the Divine — the universe of delight. Mood killer gadgets, light candles or incense and assemble any extraordinary deals with chocolates or berries. Decontaminate yourself by showering and dressing in something stunning; purge your space by cleaning up and taking care of the clothing heaps. It's additionally best to skip or go light on the substances to be completely present.

2. Soul or eye gazing.

Similarly, as with yoga, tantra starts with and bases on the breath. Picture that you're pushing the breath down through your pelvis, knees, and floor. Practice the tummy breathing strategy a few times before you bring it into sex with the goal that it turns out to be more programmed

In the ground-breaking look of your mate, there is no place to cover up, and you practice completely uncovering yourself to the next with all that you feel and all that you are. You see them completely while simultaneously leaving yourself alone observed.

Eye-to-eye connection will help both of you feel nearer during sex. Zero in on one another. Generally, this is done by investigating their left eye; however, you can investigate both if that is more agreeable to you.

Sit up straight on a cushion or seat, looking at your spouse. You can look left eye to left eye or simply look delicately at the two eyes, and you can likewise clasp hands if you like. Let the adoration that is in your heart sparkle out through your eyes. Looking at your cherished, see the awesome sparkle in their eyes, wondering about the unadulterated life power that is enlivening them. Feel the holiness of this straightforward second together. Go after two minutes. Notice what feelings or sensations come up, or on the off chance that you feel enticed to turn away. It is anything but a gazing challenge, so you can generally close your eyes for a couple of moments and afterward open them once more.

3. Hands-on hearts circuit.

The hands-on heart circuit can frequently stream pleasantly after eye staring. While sitting, confronting each other with a delicate look, carry your hands to your own heart and inhale up into your heart. As you feel the adoration that is gushing in your heart for your spouse, reach across and place the right hand on your mate's heart (with assent), and they can do the same with their right hand. Every individual's left hand at that point covers the hand that is placed on their own heart. Synchronize your breathing with moderate, profound, supporting breaths. On the breathe in, get breath and love into your own heart, and on the breath out, send that adoration from your heart down your correct arm and into your spouse's heart, making a circuit of affection and energy streaming between you. Do this for around 10 breaths.

4. Tantric massage.

This is another incredible piece of tantric sex that can be the way into numerous climaxes for the two individuals.

In this massage, one spouse gets to simply lie back and get, finding the opportunity to tune into their pleasure and sexual energy and perceive how it needs to open up through their body, while the other mate moves their hands gradually and thoughtfully along their body to let them feel each and every new sensation.

5. The yab-yum position.

This exemplary tantric sex position speaks to the association of Shiva and Shakti, the two heavenly energies of male and female.

However, recall these are simply energies, and it doesn't make a difference the sex of the members.

In any event, for connections between cis men and cis ladies, it's incredible to work on exchanging between every job.

- The base spouse (speaking of Shiva, who is vivaciously or actually penetrative) sits with folded legs on a pad in the "holding" position while the other spouse (speaking of Shakti, who is vigorously or truly responsive) can either wrap their legs over their mate's legs with their butt on the bed or a cushion or can completely sit in the lap of their spouse. The base spouse's arms should circumvent the midriff of the other spouse, whose arms circumvent the shoulders of the base mate. Your heads can be up close, or you can contact brow to temple. This position adjusts the chakras of the spouses and takes into account sexual energy to move upward along the spine.

- Once you come into an arrangement, start by taking a couple of profound, slow breaths together, synchronizing and relaxing. At that point, start to move together in moderate undulations, angling, twirling around and around; finding a stream and a musicality that feels delectable, initiating your sexual energy together. The base spouse "gives" to the mate on top who is "getting" that energy up into their body.

- Connect with your breath to grow the joy and sexual energy all through the whole body, illuminating each cell with that life power. You can have a go at remaining with more modest, inconspicuous developments, or get as lively as you can imagine; however, in any case, utilize your breath to draw orgasmic energy from your pelvis up the spine and up to your third eye (the spot between your eyebrows) or crown (the highest point of the head) and past.

- This position can be rehearsed completely dressed, bare, or in whatever way you like. You can even figure out how to have full-body energy climaxes — with no entrance at all — while remaining completely dressed; however, that may take somewhat more practice!

Tantric Massage

Tantric back massage is a happily invigorating encounter that each man and lady ought to appreciate. In addition to the fact that it feels great, there are numerous advantages related to the antiquated act of tantra that is all the more distinctly felt with customary use. Tantric back massage is a style of back massage or bodywork that draws on the standards of tantra, an old religious work starting in Central and Southeast Asia. In most advanced practice in the West, tantric back massage includes rubbing and animating the full body with a specific spotlight on delicate zones like the penis and vulva. It's occasionally alluded to as just a suggestive back massage, albeit a tantra massage additionally joins breathwork, reflection, and care components and isn't really sexual. Tantric back massage additionally has a profound and vigorous part, wherein the specialist or provider helps move the collector's energy all through the body to advance inward recuperating.

Benefits of Tantric Massage

It Enhances You Physically

The tantric back massage starts with an all-over body massage. Notably, back massage carries immense advantages to the body, for example, stimulation of the lymphatic frameworks to deplete away poisons, easing a throbbing painfulness in muscles and connective tissues, relaxing a strained body, and reducing torment.

The tantric joy that outcomes in delivery diminish pulse for people, and in men, normal discharge frees the prostate organ from developing liquids that can prompt issues. This can be accomplished through prostate back massage as well.

It Enhances You Mentally

Psychological wellness is significant, and tantric delights de-stress even the most on edge individual. This is because the joy hormone dopamine and the joy hormone oxytocin are delivered through actual touch from someone else. Contact is likewise an extraordinary tension reliever — from embraces to massage, we as a whole vibe better after adoring contact.

Consistently, tantric back massage de-focuses on the psyche to empower rest, battle sleep deprivation, gloom, and the nerves of occupied life. At the point when you are less focused on, you perform better grinding away and at home. Your emotional prosperity is critical to your wellbeing, and men specifically regularly disregard it. Standard de-focusing tantric back massage prompts unwinding and more noteworthy joy.

You Will Enjoy It

Everybody needs something to appreciate, regardless of whether it's a leisure activity, occasion, or a mitigating tantric back massage. Booking a customary tantric back massage implies there's something to anticipate. Contemplating the delight, you'll get helps your disposition.

At that point, there's the energizing expectation of voyaging or hanging tight for the doorbell, trailed by your happy tantric back massage.

At the point when it's over, you'll feel re-charged, glad, and loose with the information you'll be doing it again soon. Standard back massage also allows you to know your masseuse, making a back massage more pleasurable. Believing somebody to put their hands everywhere on your body requires some investment, and with ordinary gatherings, you'll quickly unwind and appreciate their conversation.

It Improves Your Sex Life

Tantric back massage can assist you with understanding your body through touch. A few men discover portions of them stir that they never knew existed, and surrendering control of your body is elating. As you find out about your body's response, you'll find out about your sexuality.

Figuring out how to contact and be contacted can improve your sexual coexistence at home. Back massage, situating, and seeing how the way toward uncovering and contacting is similarly as pleasurable as the closure can get you out of a homegrown trench.

Improve Your Confidence

People who experience issues with contact and sexual articulation can discover normal tantric back massage encourages them massively. Untimely discharge can be managed; however, breathing and standard exotic back massage. When you have the certainty to uncover and put your body in someone else's hands, your trust in the room will improve.

Trust in the room prompts trust in all parts of your life. Confidence is basic; without it, we consider ourselves less and don't accomplish what we are prepared to do. Tantric back massage can genuinely help your confidence.

The physical and emotional well-being advantages of tantric back massage are definitely reason enough to appreciate them consistently. Consider it a compensation for trying sincerely and an approach to remain fit, sound, and de-focused in a bustling world.

Step-by-Step Instructions for Giving a Tantric Massage

Before endeavoring to give a tantric back massage, it's useful to become familiar with a tad about tantric standards all in all, as it'll guarantee you're moving toward the experience from the point of view of sacrosanct association and purposeful joy.

- For the beneficiary, having the option to get delighted without feeling constrained to respond.

- For the provider, being eager to give delight without the need of the equivalent consequently.

- For the supplier, figuring out how to peruse the spouse's non-verbal communication and understanding the significance of touch.

- For both, overlooking time.

- Each spouse wanting to please the other.

- Strong individual cleanliness in anticipation of the experience.

It's frequently hard for somebody to communicate how one needs to be contacted, and the number of individuals is awkward in the manner they contact each other. Contacting somebody in a way that they need to be contacted requires some investment, experience, and receptiveness.

The following are guidelines for explicit sorts of tantra massage. You can do these with a mate or without help from anyone else.

Lingam Massage

A lingam massage center around regarding and giving pleasure to the penis:

1.   Get the man loose, lying on his back comfortably with their legs separated and knees twisted. Remind them to inhale profoundly all through the experience.

2.   Practice taking in their energy of excitement as you breathe in and sending them cherishing energy as you breathe out.

3.   Lubricate and massage the territories of the penis, beginning by sliding your hands up their thighs, pubic bone, and perineum.

4.   Gently, gradually rub the balls. You can pull them somewhat, cup them in your grasp to stroke them, or utilize your fingernails tenderly on them.

5.   Massage the shaft, differing your grasp, stroke groupings, and bending movements. Switch from one hand to two and from slow to quick.

6.   Don't let them peak. Keep them at the edge of climax, otherwise called edging.

7.   If they're okay with it, animate their holy spot, otherwise called the prostate.

8.   When they're prepared, permit your spouse to peak with a discharge climax.

Yoni Massage

A yoni massage centers around respecting and giving pleasure to the vulva:

1.   Have the woman lie on her back comfortably with a cushion under her hips, with knees up, grounded feet.

2.   Guide them in interfacing with their breath.

3.   Warm up with a body massage or tantric bosom massage to gradually fabricate excitement.

4.   Move to the vulva and start animating the clitoris, switching back and forth between orbiting, pushing and pulling, pulling and moving, tapping, and G-spot rub.

5.   Encourage your spouse to work on edging or to lean in to encounter different floods of climaxes.

Tantric Bosom Massage

The tantric bosom or nipple massage essentially applies tantra massage standards to the bosoms:

1.   Set the scene with candles, incense, or music that causes your mate to feel attractive.

2.   Remind them to zero in on their breath, taking long, full breaths all through the experience.

3.   Drip some oil at the focal point of their heart between the bosoms, just as over the gut.

4.   Start by rubbing the tummy to work up sexual energy before proceeding onward to the bosoms.

5.   Circle the bosoms utilizing a quill-like touch; at that point, move to rubbing and pressing them.

6.   Once their body is asking for it, move to the nipples utilizing following, squeezing, and rolling.

7.   As they approach climax, rub their body up to the neck, head, and scalp. Have them undulate their spine and rock their hips to make excitement all through the entire body, making influxes of delight.

CHAPTER 6:

How to Last Longer

A solid sexual coexistence can build your certainty, diminish pressure, and assist you with dozing better around evening time. Yet, issues with endurance or other sexual execution issues can be both disappointing and humiliating. Professionally prescribed medications can help improve erection quality and sexual execution by expanding the bloodstream to the penis. Remedy erectile capacity drugs include vardenafil (Levitra), tadalafil (Cialis), sildenafil (Viagra), and Roman ED. Yet, similarly as with every physician-endorsed drug, they accompany a few dangers. Erectile brokenness medications can prompt flushing, migraines, visual changes, vexed stomach, and nasal clog. Likewise, they can have hazardous impacts on men taking nitrate medications, blood thinners, or those with heart issues and diabetes. The porno business regularly portrays sex continuing for quite a long time, which can give a bogus thought of how long sex should last. As per a recent report led across five nations, vaginal sex, by and large, goes on for around 5 to 6 minutes. Nonetheless, there's no right measure of time for sex to last, and it's up to you and your spouse to choose what works best.

Causes of Premature Ejaculation

Why you probably won't be enduring as long as you need to. It's regular for men to complete excessively fast every so often, yet on the off chance that you almost consistently discharge after not exactly a moment of sex, you might be determined to have premature discharge.

- Psychology: Though the specific reason isn't notable, there are certain mental angles to premature discharge. Studies show that uneasiness, especially tension about your sexual execution, is connected to premature discharge. Feeling discouraged, worried, or blameworthy can likewise make you bound to complete rapidly. Men may likewise encounter premature discharge at higher rates on the off chance that they have helpless self-perception or are casualties of sexual maltreatment.

- Experience: Your degree of sexual experience can likewise influence how long you rearward in bed. Men may likewise peak quicker on the off chance that they are not having intercourse regularly, or this is their first time taking part in any sexual behavior.

- High testosterone level: Studies show that men with the premature discharge will, in general, have more significant levels of free testosterone, which can prompt side effects like loss of energy and low sex drive. In any case, researchers state that more examination is expected to decide why this is the situation.

- Hyperthyroidism: Premature discharge can likewise be brought about by hyperthyroidism, a condition wherein the thyroid organ in your neck delivers an, over the top, a hormone called thyroxine. Scientists aren't sure why thyroid issues influence your sex endurance, yet in the wake of being treated for hypothyroidism, men are significantly less liable to encounter untimely discharge.

Normal arrangements may not present similar dangers or medication communications, and a few, for example, the initial two, may really improve in general wellbeing.

1. Condoms

Since premature discharge might be a consequence of extreme touchiness, utilizing a condom is a basic arrangement that may make sex last more. The condom frames an obstruction around the penis that dulls sensation and may prompt postponed discharge.

2. The interruption and squeezing technique

Known popularly as the pause-squeeze technique, it should be possible while having intercourse or stroking off, and it includes: Having sex until you feel that you are going to discharge. Then, pulling out and crushing the tip of your penis for a few seconds, or until the need to discharge passes. And at last, proceeding to engage in sexual relations and rehashing the method when the need arises.

The hypothesis is you stop the stream, allowed the penis to rest, and afterward return to it. This can be one of the more troublesome methods for treating premature discharge since it takes a ton of discretion. Rehearsing more than once and discussing obviously with your spouse may help facilitate the cycle. Over the long run, you might have the option to prepare your body to defer discharge without having to squeeze.

3. Pelvic floor workouts

Your pelvic floor muscles are located just beneath the prostate and rectum, and simply like different muscles, they can be fortified through exercise. Specialists accept that if pelvic floor muscles are excessively feeble, it very well might be more difficult for you to defer your discharge.

To utilize your pelvic floor muscles, go about as though you are attempting to prevent yourself from peeing or passing gas and feel which muscles move. To condition these muscles, you ought to follow these means: Tighten the pelvic floor muscles — you can rest or sit if this makes it simpler. Hold the muscles tight for 3 seconds. Relax the muscles for 3 seconds. Repeat the activity the same number of times, varying. To get great outcomes, you should attempt to complete 3 arrangements of 10 redundancies every day. If you are as yet battling with completing too soon, your medical services supplier can support you or allude you to another master medical care supplier since there are additionally a few drugs or systems that you may profit by.

4. Desensitizing drugs

Desensitizing drugs use fixings like prilocaine and lidocaine, which work by impeding the nerve flags that cause you to feel delighted and torment. These meds, by and large, come as creams or splashes, and when they are applied to your penis, you will have diminished affectability and are endorsed for use in untimely discharge.

Desensitizing creams or splashes should be applied to the penis 20 to 30 minutes before sex. Since sexual delight will feel less serious, you might have the option to postpone your discharge.

There are a few downsides to this technique, nonetheless, as the prescription can likewise diminish your mate's affectability to delight. Ensure your spouse realizes you are utilizing it — as a heads up — and furthermore to ensure they don't have a set of experiences or unfavorably susceptible response or issue with its utilization.

5. Stop Smoking

Smoking could be at fault for your sexual brokenness — also a great danger of disease and horrendous breath. Smoking can hinder course, increment your danger of experiencing erectile brokenness, and decline your sperm tally and suitability.

6. Get Fit

Being overweight and neglecting to exercise can both affect your sexual exhibition, so get going and get sound. By adjusting your cardiovascular wellbeing, you could be structure room perseverance also. Be that as it may, cease from riding a bicycle excessively, as the narrowing brought about by a bike seat may cause brief erectile brokenness.

7. Needle therapy

Needle therapy is a treatment strategy for customary Chinese medication that has been polished for over 2,500 years. The act of embeddings little needles into specific focuses over the body is said to animate the sensory system and influence normal narcotics and hormones.

8. Consume more zinc

Zinc is found in numerous home grown male upgrade supplements and in light of current circumstances. Zinc insufficiency can prompt sexual brokenness and diminished testosterone levels. Yet, an excessive amount of zinc isn't beneficial for you by the same token. As opposed to enhancing, you may discover your zinc levels are best directed by eating nourishments rich in significant minerals; for example, meat, oyster, fortified breakfast grains, etc.

9. Increase L-arginine Consumption

Amino acids are the structure squares of protein. L-arginine is a fundamental amino corrosive that can be changed over to nitric oxide, which can help loosen up the veins of the penis and increment blood stream and erection quality. It acts much similar to current doctor prescribed medications do. Soy and vegetables are acceptable wellsprings of L-arginine.

10. Think about Herbs

There are endless male upgrade items available. Some that are utilized in customary medication incorporate yohimbine, Korean red ginseng, epimedium, and ginkgo Biloba.

Creators of these items realize that men invest wholeheartedly in their room execution and are eager to spend as needs be. Do your exploration before using up every last cent on a homegrown "fix."

None of these enhancements have experienced thorough testing to demonstrate their advantages or their dangers. Likewise, some testing has uncovered that these enhancements contain far less dynamic fixings than detailed. Make certain to check with your primary care physician before taking enhancements or spices.

In case you're hoping to stay away from the possible dangers of physician-recommended drugs, the way of life changes above may give the best danger-free outcomes. Also, getting in shape and stopping smoking can improve your sexual ability.

KAMA SUTRA & TANTRIC SEX PICTURES POSITIONS

Edging

Edging (additionally called surfing, topping, prodding, and that's only the tip of the iceberg) is simply the act of preventing from arriving at climax right when you're on the cusp — the allegorical "edge" just before you tumble off the precipice into the sexual peak.

This training has developed stylish in sexual wellbeing conversations as a type of "better climaxes," however it's, in reality, more than 50 years old treatment for premature discharge. Basically, this implies halting sexual incitement before you come, holding up around 30 seconds, and afterward animating yourself once more, rehashing until you're prepared to climax.

It seems like a fast win for better sex, yet edging is more similar to a long-distance race. You can't race your approach to enduring longer in bed or having a superior climax, as some who practice this case.

What's more, with regards to edging, you likewise should know about the four phases of excitement. Knowing these can assist you with narrowing down when to stop and begin incitement:

- Excitement: This is when your skin begins to flush, the muscles start getting tense, your pulse gets quicker, blood begins to stream rapidly down to the penis, vagina, and clitoris. The vagina starts getting wet while the scrotum pulls out.

- Plateau: All that occurred in stage 1 gets significantly more extraordinary. You feel yourself moving consistently nearer to climax. This is where you ought to prepare to stop or hinder incitement.

- Orgasm: A progression of nerve and muscle reactions happen, bringing about a passion for happiness, adding grease in the vagina, and discharge of semen from the penis. However, when you're working on edging, this is the stage you're attempting to stay away from until prepared.

- Resolution: After the climax, tissues re-visitation of their non-stirred sizes and tones, and all your vitals standardize, as well. This is likewise the beginning of the refractory period. It's an impermanent timespan where you can't get stimulated once more. It can keep going for a couple of moments up to a couple of days or more.

The specific passion you get during these four phases isn't the equivalent for everybody, however.

On a more comprehensive level, edging can make you all the more acutely mindful of your own sexual reactions, both performance and with your spouse, carrying care into the room.

There are a few different ways to perform edging. They all follow comparative advances that include:

- Experiencing incitement to the point not long before a climax
- Stopping incitement or changing power to evade a peak
- Waiting for a brief timeframe
- Increasing incitement to the edge once more
- Repeating the means until needing to accomplish the climax

As per the International Society for Sexual Medicine, edging can build the power of climax in certain individuals. This can apply to sex with a mate or masturbation. Counting a time of edging during sex could help develop fervor and make the peak additionally fulfilling. Rehearsing the strategy for edging may likewise make it simpler to arrive at the climax.

A recent report proposes that females who jerk off are bound to accomplish climax during sex. Individuals who experience untimely discharge may discover edging helpful because it can expand the term of sex before the climax. At the point when somebody detects they are going to climax, they can change power. This may include easing back down, evolving position, or halting incitement completely.

Expanding the span of sexual behavior can likewise change the elements by moving the concentration away from the climax. This may permit individuals to spend longer appreciating the cycle of incitement. Edging can likewise assist individuals with finding their sexual triggers without climaxing excessively fast. A recent report found that while ladies can arrive at climax through sex alone, clitoral incitement was bound to bring about climax and improved the climax.

Edging can permit open doors for individuals to attempt new exercises and methods of contacting or invigorating. It can likewise help individuals to experience with each other.

Sex is, at times, a troublesome encounter for new couples. Edging gives occasions to individuals to examine their sexual advantages and find out about one another. Studies have additionally discovered proof that successive discharge for the duration of grown-up life may assist with forestalling prostate disease.

CPSIA information can be obtained
at www.ICGtesting.com
Printed in the USA
LVHW010713151021
700520LV00009B/228